Gill Martin is a practising aromatherapist and has been a full member of the International Federation of Aromatherapists since 1987. She has worked in private practice as an aromatherapist at a sports centre and a local swimming pool. She has also worked for the Body Shop International plc as a trainer, running aromatherapy and massage workshops and other courses for staff in the UK and overseas.

Currently she runs her aromatherapy practice from home, which she combines with freelance training and looking after her daughter, Aisling.

AROMATHERAPY

An introductory guide to professional and home use

Gill Martin

Illustrated by
Shaun Williams

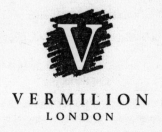

VERMILION
LONDON

First published by Macdonald Optima in 1989

1 3 5 7 9 10 8 6 4 2

This revised edition published in the United Kingdom in
1996 by Vermilion
an imprint of Ebury Press
Random House UK Ltd
Random House
20 Vauxhall Bridge Road
London SW1V 2SA

Random House Australia (Pty) Ltd
20 Alfred Street, Milsons Point, Sydney,
New South Wales 2061, Australia

Random House New Zealand Limited
18 Poland Road, Glenfield,
Auckland 10, New Zealand

Random House, South Africa (Pty) Limited
PO Box 337, Bergvlei, South Africa

Random House UK Limited Reg. No. 954009

A CIP catalogue record for this book is available from the
British Library.

ISBN 0 09 181276 3

Typeset in Sabon by Deltatype Ltd, Ellesmere Port,
Cheshire
Printed and bound in Great Britain by Mackays of
Chatham, plc

Papers used by Vermilion are natural, recyclable products
made from wood grown in sustainable forests.

CONTENTS

FOREWORD

The premise is irresistible – aromatherapy is an extremely pleasant way to relax or refresh yourself using essential oils extracted from plants. The ancients knew all about it, but we somehow lost the knack. That is one reason why I am grateful for a book like this. It arrives as an invaluable refresher course, reminding us of the benefits of aromatherapy at a time when the world is throwing any number of new stresses at us.

Aromatherapy is a very effective riposte to those stresses – so effective, in fact, that its components need to be handled knowledgeably and with care, which is why some people may feel more comfortable relying on professional aromatherapists. A major advantage of Gill Martin's research is that she comprehensively covers both professional and personal use, emphasizing the ease of aromatherapy without downplaying the care you should take if you are using essential oils at home.

I've already said that aromatherapy is irresistible. For me at least part of the reason is that it is still something of a mystery. Science only partially explains aromatherapy's potency. Its power also makes an appeal to the spirit. Consider my answer to jet lag. It's a permanent threat for me because I spend so much of the year travelling for The Body Shop. The minute I get where I'm going, I usually jump in a bath with some relaxing essential oils and soak for a while. Then, when I get out, I leave the water in the tub with the bathroom door open so that my room becomes suffused with fragrance. At that particular moment, I don't care about the hows and whys of aromatherapy. All I need to know is that my little ritual will work to lift my mood. And it *does* work – *every time*.

Anita Roddick, O.B.E.
Founder and Chief Executive of the Body Shop

1

WHAT IS AROMATHERAPY?

Aromatherapy is a therapeutic treatment combining massage and essential oils to enhance well-being, restore balance and treat a variety of conditions. It is a natural method of healing with the pure aromatic substances and the nurturing touch of the therapist encouraging the body's own healing powers.

ANCIENT ORIGINS

Although the word 'aromatherapy' was not used until the beginning of this century, the use of aromatic plants is as old as human life. Our ancient ancestors soon discovered which would aid digestion, which would cure diarrhoea and used the plants around them to treat various health problems. Their sense of smell was probably more acute than ours; it was vital when hunting or avoiding the enemy and had not been deadened by the polluted atmosphere of today. They would use this when choosing plants, though the scent would be more noticeable when aromatic substances were burned, either when cooking food or when used as firewood. Through burning plants other properties were also discovered. The smoke might make the whole group feel sleepy or full of life and often special powers would be attributed to a particular herb. Burning plants became associated with rituals and magic, indeed 'smoking' was used to drive out evil spirits.

The use of aromatics also played an important part in the ancient civilizations of Egypt, Babylon, Greece and Rome. Though advanced in many ways, none of these peoples are thought to have developed a way of distilling the essential oils

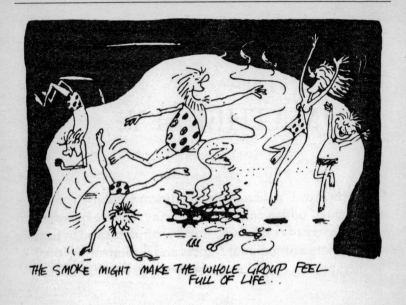

THE SMOKE MIGHT MAKE THE WHOLE GROUP FEEL
FULL OF LIFE.

from the various herbs, trees and flowers. Most of the oils they used were infusions of fragrant substances in fatty oils, most notably in castor oil in Egypt and olive oil in Greece.

These ointments and oils were used for both medicinal and cosmetic purposes. On uncovering tombs in the pyramids, archaeologists have found various pots and jars made of alabaster or glass containing unguents still smelling of frankincense and myrrh, while clay tablets show how cedarwood oil was used for mummification as well as in hair and body preparations. The ancient Greeks made use of the medical knowledge of the Egyptians as well as making their own discoveries about aromatic plants. In turn the Greeks passed on much of their expertise to the Romans.

In the West we are only just beginning to rediscover the value of natural medicine, but in India and China here is an unbroken tradition dating back to before 2,000 BC. In India, ancient origins form the basis of the Ayurvedic medicine used today, while in China herbal medicine and acupuncture have run side by side since the days of the Yellow Emperor around 2,500 BC.

FIRST DISTILLATIONS OF ESSENTIAL OILS

Through the translation of Greek and Roman books, medical knowledge built up over thousands of years passed to the Arab world. It was here that essential oils were first distilled towards the end of the tenth century AD. The discovery of a method of distillation which has changed very little even today, is attributed to a physician known as Avicenna. The first essential oil to be obtained this way was oil of rose and records show that lavender, camomile and camphor oils were also in use.

Back in Europe little is known of the progress of herbal medicine during what is known historically as the Dark Ages. It wasn't until the twelfth century that we know crusading knights began to bring back essences from Arabia. They also learnt the methods of production and so soon essences from native plants such as lavender, rosemary and basil were added to the precious flower oils such as rose and jasmine. The use of herbs and essential oils began to flourish. The knowledge was made widely available in the form of famous herbals such as those by Gerarde and Culpeper. Posies of aromatic plants were used to ward off infection, rooms were strewn with herbs and large households even had their own stills for the production of essential oils.

The use of essential oils continued throughout the seventeenth and eighteenth centuries, mainly now by ordinary people in the home using skills passed on from generation to generation. A few essential oils such as peppermint, clove, lavender and camphor can still be found in pharmacopiea of today, though many others fell out of use as modern medicine developed.

Until the early twentieth century, essential oils had always been classed along with herbal remedies or valued for their cosmetic use. In the early 1920s Renée Gattefossé, a chemist in a French perfume company, became interested in and did much research into the medicinal properties of essential oils. There is a famous story of how on burning his hand he plunged it into neat lavender oil and to his surprise not only did the wound heal amazingly quickly but it also left no scarring. His book *Aromatherapie* was published in 1928.

The pioneers of aromatherapy came in the main part from France. Following Gattefossé came Dr Jean Valnet, a French army surgeon who used essential oils extensively during the French Indo-China war in treating battle wounds. He also undertook work in psychiatric hospitals using the oils with mentally disturbed patients. His book *Aromatherapie* published in 1964 is available in translation as *The Practice of Aromatherapy*. It is the classic text book for all serious practitioners of aromatherapy.

Around the same time as Dr Valnet, Mme Marguerite Maury was taking a different line of approach in her work with essential oils. She was a biochemist not a doctor, and used the oils externally for therapeutic and cosmetic purposes. She developed the basis of a therapy using a combination of essential oils and massage, a tradition carried on by many aromatherapists today.

The interest in aromatherapy in Britain is fairly recent. Towards the end of her life Mme Maury moved to England and two of her assistants still have well-known practices in London. In 1977 the first English work on aromatherapy, *The Art of Aromatherapy* by Robert Tisserand, was published. The shelves are now full with books on all aspects of the subject from aromantics to aromatherapy for veterinary use! There are over 80 establishments teaching courses in aromatherapy and the number of qualified aromatherapists has soared. There are many aromatherapy associations and 1991 saw the formation of the Aromatherapy Organizations Council (AOC), the governing body for the profession in the UK.

NATURAL VERSUS SYNTHETIC

The essential oils used in aromatherapy are pure, natural substances which do not produce side-effects and are non-habit forming. Unfortunately this cannot always be said about conventional medicine. Though essential oils are

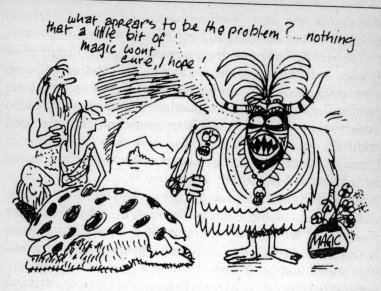

simple substances in terms of their molecular structure, they are complex in terms of the number of active constituents that make up each particular essence (see Chapter 2). As in any holistic therapy the maxim 'The whole is greater than the sum of the constituent parts' applies to aromatherapy.

When our ancestors used aromatic plants, their healing properties were put down to magic qualities. It wasn't until the nineteenth century that experimental chemists began looking in depth at various medicinal plants and succeeded in isolating their therapeutically active substances. Soon these isolated constituents began to be used in preference to the whole, natural plant or essence. Shortly after, towards the end of the nineteenth century, they were being produced synthetically in the laboratory and natural medicines fell out of use in favour of these new, modern drugs. Today the range of synthetic drugs is vast, with the major pharmaceutical companies trying to win over the consumer with their latest headache cure, or to convince doctors that their products are better than those of their rivals.

Medical science maintains that if the chemical formula of a synthetic drug is similar to that of a natural one then the body will accept it in the same way. In the aromatherapists' view this is not the case. With a natural substance, the body recognizes it as friendly, will use what it needs and pass the rest away. An artificial drug, however, will be identified as foreign and treated in the same way as invading bacteria. Over millions of years our bodies have adapted to the natural food and medicines found around us. It is too short a time to expect them to adapt to synthetic drugs and chemical food additives. So though a particular drug may be effective in treating a condition, it may also produce side-effects as the body tries hard to detoxify itself.

Side-effects in modern medicines are also the result of using isolated active constituents rather than the whole plant. An essential oil will contain a large number of principles which balance and enhance each other. Chemists may take one constituent and use it alone to treat a particular symptoms, yet without the other parts of the plant the balance is lost and unwanted side-effects can occur. It still needs to be said, however, that while essential oils are safe in the hands of a qualified therapist, they are very concentrated and potent materials which should always be treated with care.

DRUG DEPENDENCY

A further problem of chemically synthesized drugs is that the body will become habituated to them. At first one sleeping pill will have the desired effect, then as the body gets used to that two will be necessary. Similarly, with long-term use of laxatives the bowels lose their ability to function naturally.

One of the most common examples of drug dependency is the use of tranquillizers and anti-depressants. The body responds to these as it would to nicotine, caffeine or heroin and the taker becomes addicted. Severe withdrawal symptoms can occur and it is usually the people who resorted to tranquillizers in the first place who are least able to cope with them. Thus the body can become addicted to a substance whose effects are diminishing, so the dose is increased and the vicious circle completed.

TREATING THE WHOLE PERSON

Surrounded by such an array of medication, it is now the norm to run for the aspirin bottle at the first sign of a cold or headache. Similarly many people are not happy if they leave the doctor's surgery without a prescription. However, immediately removing the symptoms doesn't lead us to the original cause of the complaint. A headache may have many causes – tension in the neck, lack of sleep, a hangover. Removing the pain may allow us to carry on when the body is trying to tell us to rest. With a hangover the body is telling us it didn't like what we did to it and needs time to remove its toxins, not to be given more. We often catch a cold when we're feeling run down and need a rest but instead of doing so we pump ourselves with chemicals and carry on. In the end the cold lasts a lot longer and leaves us feeling even more drained. Tranquillizers and anti-depressants may help in the short term but the problem cauing the anxiety or depression will still be there.

When working with a client, an aromatherapist will not just treat a symptom but look for the possible causes. He or she will also look at the whole person.

THE ROLE OF THE AROMATHERAPIST

Having seen some of the drawbacks of modern medicine, it is necessary at this point to say that the aromatherapist does not claim to be able to perform all the functions of a fully trained doctor. Though there is little doubt that essential oils can, for example, be more effective in fighting infection than antibiotics, the use of plant essences for serious conditions is limited either to herbalists or aromatherapists with a strong medical training (see Chapter 7). The majority of aromatherapists deal with non life-threatening conditions – minor ailments, skin problems and in particular stress or emotional difficulties. A client with more serious problems will be referred to a doctor, herbalist or homeopath depending on preference. Aromatherapy can still be used in most cases in conjunction

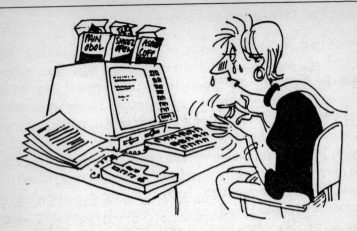

WE OFTEN CATCH A COLD WHEN WE'RE FEELING RUN DOWN
AND NEED A REST BUT INSTEAD OF DOING SO WE PUMP
OURSELVES FULL OF CHEMICALS AND CARRY ON.

with these other forms of healthcare and thus can truly be seen
as a complementary therapy. It is also a valuable preventative
therapy which, by keeping a client well balanced emotionally
and physically, reduces the chances of serious illness occurring.

A further distinction needs to be made between a trained
aromatherapist and a beauty therapist using products with
essential oils. The latter may advertise aromatherapy treatment but will often use a ready blended oil to treat a particular
condition, without looking at the whole person. Though it is
good to see a return to the use of natural ingredients,
including essential oils, in cosmetics and beauty products, it is
also necessary to see the broader scope of aromatherapy as a
holistic treatment.

2
HOW DOES AROMATHERAPY WORK?

The main tools of the aromatherapist are essential oils, and before explaining how they work it is necessary to know what they are and where they come from.

WHAT ARE ESSENTIAL OILS?

Essential oils are pure aromatic substances extracted or distilled from flowers, trees, fruits and herbs. They contain all the special properties of the plant including its odour. They are often thought of as being the life-force of the plant, the part of the plant which sums up the whole. The properties of the plant are not lost in the extraction process but in some way are concentrated and even enhanced. Thus essential oils are very powerful and need only be used in very small quantities. Essential oils are not fatty, some are very light and more like alcohol, a substance in which the oils will dissolve. They vary considerably in odour intensity and the rate at which they evaporate. Many are extremely volatile and they are usually stored in dark glass air-tight bottles to avoid deterioration.

All parts of a plant can be used to obtain essential oil, and in some cases different parts of the same plant produce different essences. From the orange tree, for example, we get orange oil from the rind of the fruit, petitgrain from the leaves and neroli from the blossom. The therapeutic value of each of these oils is different.

HOW ESSENTIAL OILS ARE EXTRACTED

Coming as they do from a range of different plants, fruits and flowers essential oils are extracted in a variety of different ways. Aromatic plants produce oils in special cells. These may be near the surface or within the secretory glands or ducts. Different plants also produce different quantities of oil and these two factors determine the method and ease of extraction as well as the amount of essential oil obtained.

The easiest method of extraction is by *simple pressure*, which is confined to the citrus fruit family. Orange, lemon, grapefruit, mandarin and bergamot are among those used in aromatherapy. The best quality oils are obtained by hand pressure though now most manufacturers use machines.

The most common method of extracting essential oils used today is *steam distillation*, a method familiar to most of us from our school chemistry days. The plant is held over boiling water and the steam produced draws off the essential oil. The steam is collected and cooled forming water in which the essential oil will either float or sink depending on its density. The water is then drawn off leaving only the essential oil. This oil from the *first* distillation is the best quality. The water can be re-used several times producing second, third and even fourth distillations. Essences obtained by this method include many of the commonly used ones such as lavender, rosemary, clary sage and peppermint. A cruder method of distillation involves heating the plant in water instead of above steam, producing an inferior quality oil. It is also possible to carry out the process in a vacuum where steam will be produced at a lower temperature, giving an even finer oil.

Some of the flower oils are extracted by a more complex process known as *enfleurage*. The flower heads are pressed in layers of purified fat and left until the essential oil has been removed and absorbed by the fat. As the flowers wilt they are replaced by new ones, this continuing until the fat is saturated with essential oil. This fatty compound is known as a *pommade* and was often used as an ointment or perfume. Now it is more common to continue the process and remove the essential oil from the fat. This is done by mixing the pommade with alcohol, in which the essential oil dissolves but the fat is insoluble. The alcohol is then evaporated off by gentle heating, leaving the pure essential oil in the container.

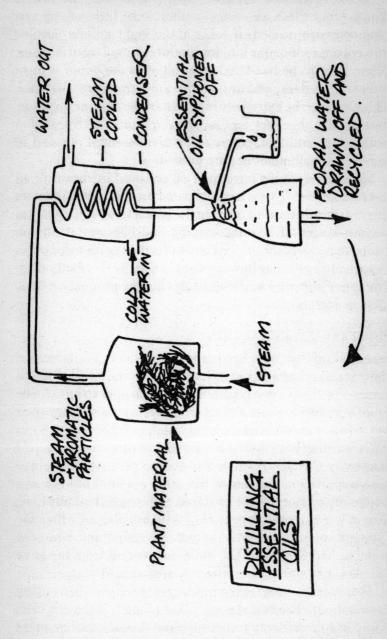

WATER OUT

STEAM COOLED

CONDENSER

ESSENTIAL OIL SYPHONED OFF

FLORAL WATER DRAWN OFF AND RECYCLED.

COLD WATER IN

STEAM + AROMATIC PARTICLES

STEAM

PLANT MATERIAL

DISTILLING ESSENTIAL OILS

Oils obtained in this way are known as *absolutes*. The flowers which yield these absolutes contain very little oil so vast quantities are needed. It takes about eight million jasmine flowers to produce one kilogramme of essential oil of jasmine. These have to be hand picked at night as the odour is most intense after dark, and also before the flowers are a day old. This explains the extremely high cost of the jasmine absolute. Fortunately absolutes tend to be even more concentrated in both odour and therapeutic value than essential oils and so only very small quantities are needed.

Some flowers now have their oil removed by means of an *organic solvent*. This is a complicated process which involves mixing the flowers in solvent to extract the oil, then via various stages of heating, cooling and filtering, alcohol is added to dissolve the oil. The alcohol is then evaporated off as described above. The flower oils produced by this method are not as fine a quality as the absolutes but the production costs are considerably less.

PURITY OF ESSENTIAL OILS

Essential oils are now becoming more widely available and there is a dazzling array of different producers, packaging and prices. For the lay person, knowing which ones to buy can be quite a problem. Most serious aromatherapists will buy their oils direct from suppliers by mail order, or in specialist shops. After working with the oils for a while the therapist develops a sensitivity towards them and is able to perceive differences between different bottles of the same essential oil. No two bottles of marjoram, for example, will smell the same. The aroma will not only depend on purity but also on where the aromatic plant grew when it was harvested and what the weather had been like. The same essential oil from the same supplier may smell quite different from year to year.

There are, however, a few guidelines to follow when buying essential oils. The first is price. Unfortunately if the oils seem cheap in comparison to other suppliers then the quality won't be as good. There simply aren't short cuts to producing good quality essential oils. Cheaper oils may be from third or fourth distillations or they may be from the wrong part of the plant. For example the best quality oil from the juniper tree is from the juniper berry. An oil produced from the leaves as well will be cheaper, but not so powerful in its therapeutic properties. The oils may also have been mixed with cheaper oils or in some cases even with synthetic oils to stretch them further. A classic example is the fact that France actually exports more lavender oil than it produces. It is usually at the level of the manufacturer or exporter that this adulteration takes place so the wholesaler or retailer may be unaware of it. This is why most serious therapists use established suppliers who know the business well and can offer a guarantee of purity.

Another point to watch for is a uniform price throughout one manufacturer's range. Due to different methods of extraction the prices of different essential oils should vary enormously. If they don't, you will either be paying over the odds for your orange oil or be buying an inferior quality sandalwood. Also make sure the oils are packaged in dark glass bottles. The effects of light will cause deterioration of the oils, so clear glass bottles are no good and plastic is even worse as the oils can attack the plastic causing contamination. Some suppliers dilute the more expensive oils such as rose or jasmine in a carrier oil to make the price accessible to more people but this should be clearly stated on the bottle.

There is a list of reputable suppliers at the back of the book, but if you discover others then spend some time talking to the stockist about them. If they know a lot about the oils and can tell you about their suppliers then, unless they are very unscrupulous, the oils will probably be all right to buy.

CHEMISTRY AND STRUCTURE OF ESSENTIAL OILS

Plants manufacture essential oils by breaking down naturally occurring elements such as carbon, oxygen and nitrogen and putting them together in different combinations to produce aromatic molecules. From a relatively small number of building blocks put together in different ways, a large number of different essential oils are produced.

The constituents of essential oils are mostly based on a

framework of carbon atoms made up in multiples of five. Onto this framework will hang atoms of other elements, producing a wide range of different aromatic molecules. These molecules are small, normally consisting of chains of around 25 or 30 carbon atoms with associated elements hanging on. This molecular simplicity is of great importance when considering how the body can absorb the oils. Other compounds may consist of chains of many thousands of atoms.

These different compounds can be put into a variety of groups such as acids, alcohol, phenols or terpenes. It is these constituents that the chemists separate and use individually. Phenols, such as eugenol and eucalyptol, are powerful antiseptics yet it has been shown that using the whole oil is more effective. A 1 per cent dilution of clove oil is three or four times more effective than its main constituent eugenol. Again we have another example of synergy, that is the co-ordination of various constituents being more active than just one part.

It is the combination of many active constituents that makes each oil unique. It also accounts for the fact that one essential oil may have a wide range of uses and also that many different oils can be used for the same condition. This often produces a certain amount of scepticism in the lay person – can one oil really treat such a variety of symptoms? Taking lavender as an example, it can be used as a pain reliever, a decongestant, a disinfectant or an anti-depressant to name just a few uses. It can be used for complaints as diverse as acne, migraine, 'flu and insomnia. Similarly a person suffering from migraine may equally well be treated using marjoram or for 'flu, tea-tree may be used. It is by working holistically that the aromatherapist will pick the right combination of oils for a particular person at a particular time.

In summary, essential oils are simple in terms of their molecular structure, yet complex in the number of active constituents which make up each individual essence. It is the combination of these constituents which give the essential oil its own distinctive aroma and range of therapeutic values. This combination will also prove more effective than any one isolated component.

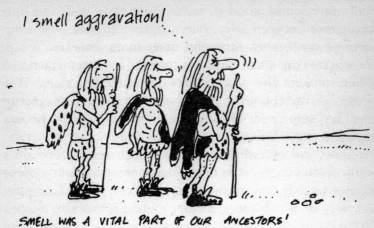

I smell aggravation!

SMELL WAS A VITAL PART OF OUR ANCESTORS' DEFENCE MECHANISM...

HOW THE BODY USES ESSENTIAL OILS

The challenge most often levelled at aromatherapy by the sceptic is 'how can just smelling something do you any good?'. There is, of course, far more to aromatherapy than that but nevertheless our sense of smell does play an important part. Today, smell is probably our most neglected sense, though to our ancestors it was a vital part of their defence mechanism. They would use it when tracking animals for food or to sense that they themselves were being hunted. Indeed our reaction to smell is actually quicker than to pain or sound.

In some way or another we cultivate our other senses. We watch television or visit an art gallery, we listen to music, we go out for a meal and we may stroke a cat or touch our partners. How often do we actually do something for the sense of smell alone? We might remark upon smells when we sense them, that of new baked bread or fresh mown hay, but only rarely do we bend down to a rose simply to enjoy its fragrance. Even perfume is often just sprayed on as the last stage in our grooming routine.

Our sense of smell, however, is more powerful than we think. In fact when we eat that meal, it is our noses which really reveal how good it 'tastes'. Our taste buds can only distinguish between salty, sweet, bitter and sour, while our sense of smell is ten thousand times more sensitive. We all come across this when we have a cold and food seems tasteless. When smokers give up cigarettes one of the first things they notice is how food tastes much better and how their sense of smell has improved. In fact, pollution has an effect on our ability to smell. Drive out of London or any other big city to the coast and everything smells so much better; food on a picnic always tastes better than it does at home. So our sense of smell is actually at work though we don't realize it. This is just one way in which our olfactory system is working for us. Think about what happens when we smell food cooking, how it makes us feel hungry, or how the smell of rotten food can make us feel sick. How often does a particular smell remind us of some past event? The perfume industry bases its marketing strategy on suggesting that a perfume will create a certain mood or that an aftershave will act as an aphrodisiac. Somehow our sense of smell is linked with a variety of things from memory to sexual arousal to digestion.

HOW THE OLFACTORY SYSTEM WORKS

Just behind the bridge of the nose is a structure called the olfactory bulb and from here the olfactory nerve cells reach down into the mucus of the nasal cavity. Extending from these nerve cells are tiny hairs known as cilia, which are excited in response to olfactory stimuli (or things that smell). This impulse passes through the nerve cells to the olfactory bulb which in turn sends the impulse directly to the brain via the olfactory tracts. The olfactory nerve tracts run into the part of the brain known as the limbic system. It is this part of the brain that is in someway tied up with memory and emotion. In addition to this, the limbic system is connected to the hypothalamus. This structure governs the pituitary gland which in turn controls the other glands and therefore our whole hormonal system. So when we smell something there is an immediate effect on our autonomic nervous system and our hormonal system. These systems are responsible for fear

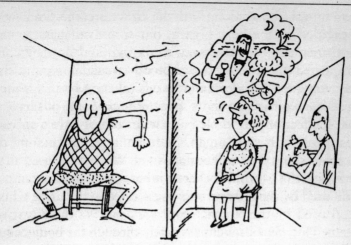

AT PRESENT WORK IS BEING DONE TO FIND OUT MORE ABOUT PHEROMONES.

and anger responses, appetite control, growth rate, sexual responses, digestion, heart rate, our reaction to stress, memory and many other responses. This not only demonstrates how important our sense of smell is but illustrates how powerful aromatherapy can be in helping with emotional problems.

We may also react to smells in an unconscious way. At present work is being done to find out more about pheromones, or odorous substances produced by the sebaceous glands of humans. Pheromones are complex substances which are thought to have an effect on those around us. They tend to be produced under the arms and around the genitals and the glands excrete more pheromones when we are frightened, excited or sexually aroused. Thus they are thought to play a part in the way people are attracted to one another or the way we can sense each other's emotions.

ABSORPTION INTO THE BLOODSTREAM

Our olfactory system is not the only one activated when we smell something, such as an essential oil. The aromatic molecules will have evaporated into the air and can be taken down into the lungs along with the air we breathe. Some will be exhaled in the next breath, but some will pass to the bloodstream in the same way as oxygen and nutrients are transported around the body. Blood circulates around the body very rapidly indeed and so oils taken in by this means can have an effect in a short space of time. Some oils have a general effect on the whole body while others have a special affinity for a particular organ. On reaching this organ some or all of the essential oil will be deposited. When it has used all it needs then the organ will excrete what is left. So for example an oil used by the kidneys will be excreted in the urine while an oil used by the stomach will pass out via the digestive system. Thus the oils will pass safely through the body being used as the body needs them.

The second way of getting essential oils into the bloodstream is via the skin. Essential oils can be mixed with natural vegetable oils, creams or lotions and applied locally or over the whole body. If the molecular structure of a substance is small enough then it will be absorbed by the skin. The molecular size is of great importance in this process. As stated earlier, essential oils are of very small molecular size and so it is important that any carrier oil they are mixed in must have small molecules too. Mineral-based oils such as Vaseline or baby oil, or products containing animal fats such as lanolin sit on the surface of the skin and therefore will not aid the absorption of the essential oils.

Once the oils have passed through the skin they will be absorbed by tissue fluids, taken into the lymphatic system and from there will pass into the bloodstream to be circulated around the body. The time this takes varies from person to person, anything from around 20 minutes to several hours. Likewise the effects may last from several hours up to several days.

A third way for an essential oil to reach the bloodstream is via the digestive system. This process of absorption takes longer than by any other method as the oils pass, along with food matter, through the complex workings of the digestive system. There is a split amongst aromatherapists as to whether essential oils should ever be taken internally, as not only is transcutaneous absorption (through the skin) safer, it can also be a lot quicker (see Chapter 3).

So there are various methods by which the body receives essential oils, all varying in speed. Whichever method we use we always smell the aroma and some of the aromatic particles are always inhaled. Thus, for example, when a blend of oils is massaged into the body there is the instantaneous effect on the olfactory system and the rapid absorption through the lungs, followed by the slightly slower absorption through the skin.

HEALTHY CELLS – HEALTHY BODY

Once in the bloodstream, how does an essential oil have an effect on the body? To take an example, essential oil of rosemary has an affinity with the liver. On reaching the liver in its journey through the bloodstream, the essential oil needed will be dissolved into the tissue fluid, along with any other substances the liver needs such as oxygen and the fat-soluble vitamins. The essential oil contains a number of chemical substances that the liver cells might need to remain healthy. These simple substances can be used easily and therefore rapidly. Other organs will use the essential oil in a similar way.

Some oils, however, are less specific in their effect and act on body tissues in general. They may perform a variety of functions – stimulating, cleansing and generally toning. Their most important function is their ability to balance the body systems and improve the body's own defence mechanisms. Essential oils will also help promote healthy new cell growth; in particular neroli (orange blossom) and lavender are noted for this. Some essential oils also contain plant hormones which can either stimulate or balance the production of our hormones. Fennel for example contains oestrogen.

It is because essential oils are recognized as friendly by the body that they are so readily accepted by the cells. And a healthy body depends on healthy cells.

3

WHAT THE AROMATHERAPIST DOES

There are various ways in which the aromatherapist can use his or her basic tools, the essential oils, in treating a patient. In general a session will be centred around a massage but in some cases other methods of administering the oils will be used or advised for use at home.

INHALATIONS

Though this method could be used with any oil for any complaint, as a way of getting oil into the bloodstream, it is usually used for problems of the lungs or air passages. The aromatherapist will most likely suggest inhalations at home to back up the treatment, but sometimes they might be appropriate during a treatment session. This could be the case with a patient suffering from sinusitis where the condition is advanced and painful. An inhalation may help to loosen the trapped fluid and the antibiotic properties of the oils will help to fight the infection. This could be followed by a gentle face massage to encourage drainage and ease a headache if there is one.

An inhalation is carried out by adding a few drops of essential oil to near boiling water in a bowl. The client leans over the bowl with a towel over his or her head and takes deep breaths. Breathing through the nose will help to unblock nasal passages while breathing through the mouth will ease a sore throat. The steam in itself helps to fight infection and with the antibiotic and antiviral properties of essential oils, inhalations make an effective way of fighting a cold or 'flu. The

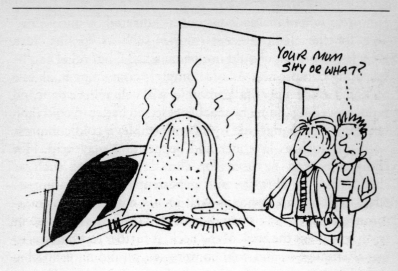

amount of time spent over the water starts with short bursts of
about 30 seconds, building up to several minutes as the client
feels more comfortable. Lavender is a good oil for colds and
can also be used to ensure a good night's sleep. Some of the
oils commonly associated with the treatment of colds, such as
eucalyptus or thyme, are most stimulating and best avoided in
the evening. Bronchitis sufferers can also benefit from
inhalations. Any phlegm will be loosened and then a gentle
massage will be comforting and help ease any tension caused
by the strain of coughing. For some skin complaints a similar
method is used to steam the face. In conditions such as acne
where massage may be painful, after thorough cleansing of
the skin a steam facial may be used instead. Some therapists
use a facial steamer for this purpose instead of the rather
crude method involving bowls and boiling water.

COMPRESSES

An aromatic compress comprises a clean cloth soaked in
either hot or cold water to which essential oils have been
added. The excess water is wrung out and the cloth applied
repeatedly to the affected area. An aromatherapist may use a

compress where massage is contra-indicated or uncomfortable for the client. Recent injuries such as sprains, torn muscles or bruises should not be massaged, but relief can be felt using compresses. A cold compress containing analgesic oils such as lavender and camomile will help relieve pain and reduce swelling. Some headaches respond better to cold than heat and where massage is uncomfortable, a cold compress with oils such as lavender and peppermint may help. Hot compresses can be used for chronic conditions such as rheumatism or fibrositis and persistent pain from injuries. Menstrual cramp responds well to hot compresses of marjoram oil and the same can be used for headaches if they stem from tension at the back of the neck. A further technique is to use alternate hot and cold compresses, an old naturopathic technique which is said to help the healing of old injuries.

BATHS

Though obviously not a part of the session, an aromatherapist will often advise aromatic baths as a back-up treatment between sessions. He or she will make up a blend of oils, ready diluted in a carrier oil for the client to use either in the morning or evening. A long soak in a warm bath before going to bed can be soothing and relaxing and, with oils such as lavender and marjoram, particularly helpful for insomnia sufferers. If your problem is getting going in the morning then a bath first thing with stimulating oils such as rosemary would be advised for you.

VAPORIZATION

Evaporating essential oils into the atmosphere can be useful either for creating a mood or fighting infection. Many aromatherapists use an oil burner in their treatment rooms before a client arrives. This can be very helpful for anxious or nervous people to help them relax before they have a massage. At home they can be used for a similar purpose – maybe the whole family would benefit from a calming, relaxing fragrance. Some essential oils, namely eucalyptus and tea-tree, contain constituents which are air-borne bacteriacides, so can be extremely useful during epidemics of 'flu, chicken-pox or measles. They also make good insect repellants and room fresheners. You can buy specially made vaporizers consisting of a container holding a candle, supporting a dish to which water and a few drops of essential oil have been added. The candle gently warms the water and oil, which evaporate producing a wonderful aroma. Other simpler methods include putting the oils into a bowl of boiling water, placing a damp cloth containing essential oils over a radiator.

INTERNAL MEDICATION

Aromatherapists can really be divided into two groups: those who advocate the use of essential oils as an internal medica-tion and those who don't. These two different schools of thought can really be traced back to two of the pioneers of modern day aromatherapy. Dr Jean Valnet and Mme Mar-guerite Maury. Jean Valnet was a qualified doctor and surgeon and one of his main interests was in the antibacterial effects of the essential oils. Oils were used internally and externally as appropriate. Mme Maury on the other hand had no medical qualifications. She was a biochemist whose interest was in the cosmetic use of the oils and their effect on mood and emotion. She concentrated entirely on the external application of essential oils, never using them as an internal medication. Thus there is a clear difference in backgrounds. Many aromatherapists in Britain do not have previous medical backgrounds (though all those who are members of the International Federation of Aromatherapists have fol-lowed a course in anatomy and physiology) and prefer to stick to the external use of the oils, with massage being an equally important part of the therapy.

Many aromatherapists are beginning to see that in many ways transcutaneous absorption (through the skin) can be more powerful than ingestion and also safer. There are several reasons for this. Firstly, the skin is the largest organ of the body and tests have shown that if necessary more oil can be absorbed through the skin in a short space of time than could be tolerated by the stomach. Secondly, essential oils are very powerful substances and if used in large quantities internally they could irritate or damage the stomach lining. There is also the possibility of toxicity when they reach the liver and kidneys. It also takes longer for the essential oils to be distributed around the body when they have to go via the digestive system. Having said this, internal usage is practised with success by medically trained doctors using aromatherapy and also by some herbalists. Those aromatherapists who do use oils internally do so in small quantities which have been well diluted. Dilution is usually done in a small amount of alcohol which is then diluted further with water, so very small quantities of essential oil are being taken at a time. Some books suggest taking the oil on sugar or honey, a practice which is now frowned upon. The sugar does not dissolve the essential oil but just makes it more palatable.

Some of the aromatherapy organizations have a policy by which their members do not use essential oils internally in the treatment of their clients. This usually reflects their bias as either medical, holistic or cosmetic aromatherapists (for more discussion see Chapter 7).

MASSAGE

Massage is an ancient healing art with an unfortunate reputation in modern society. Fortunately, it is now becoming accepted as a serious healing therapy and the variety of different types of massage grow in number all the time. Biodynamic massage, shiatsu, postural integration, rolfing and pulsing are all forms of massage but the practitioner's method of working is very different in each case.

Aromatherapy massage was developed as a means of applying the oils for the skin, but the benefits far exceed the simple absorption of the oils into the body. Massage will help ease tight muscles, improve circulation and lymph flow, help the body eliminate toxins or help ease pain in a specific area. Our natural reaction to pain is to rub or hold the hurt area, a toe stubbed on a chair feels better if we hold and rub it. Massage is an extension of this natural reaction. Massage also has a powerful effect on the mind and emotions. It can help increase awareness of our own bodies, help balance the flow of energy or release emotional tension stored in our muscles. It also provides the means for direct contact between the aromatherapist and his or her client, helping to increase communication and build up trust.

Aromatherapy massage is a combination of techniques from other massage styles, adapted to help the absorption of the essential oils and to promote a feeling of well-being for the client. No two aromatherapists will massage in the same way, nor will one aromatherapist give the same massage to all clients or even give the same massage to one client on each visit. Each massage given is unique, tailored to the specific needs of that person at that time. Each aromatherapist develops his or her own style, which will be constantly altered and adapted.

Despite the personal variations in technique, all aromatherapy massage will be smooth and flowing, without harsh or jarring movements. Stroking or *effleurage* is a movement from Swedish massage much used in aromatherapy. It consists of long, slow, gentle strokes made with the whole hand and normally directed towards the heart. The pressure can be varied, with deeper strokes affecting the muscles and circulation while lighter strokes tend to have more of an effect on the nervous system. Smooth but deeper kneading movements follow, to warm the muscles for any deeper work. At this point aromatherapy massage leaves Swedish massage and its more vigorous hacking and pounding movements – while being an excellent form of physical massage, most Swedish massage doesn't take into account the mental and emotional state of the receiver.

As a total reaction against this during the 1960s, intuitive massage became popular. The giver would 'tune in' to the receiver and use whatever touch and movement he or she felt appropriate. Though this was a wonderful way of heightening personal awareness and developing non-verbal communication, a less experienced masseur could easily miss areas of muscle spasm which needed attention. Today intuitive massage is less vague in its practice and it is now taught with various strokes to be used as and when needed.

Aromatherapy massage is based on a similar approach. The therapist aims to give the body what it needs on a physical level while still remaining nurturing and taking into account the emotional state of the receiver. Some people respond well to a fairly deep, physical massage while someone with emotional problems may need more gentle handling. Any deeper work on knotted muscles will be done gently rather than vigorously. This work can sometimes be painful and the therapist will decide just what is appropriate for each client. A small amount of discomfort might be felt in easing out a muscle spasm, but too high a degree of pain will cause the client to tense up, defeating the point of a massage. The aromatherapist will sense what a client needs, but will also ask if a massage feels all right and/or request to be told if it is too uncomfortable.

MIXING THE MASSAGE OILS

Essential oils are very concentrated substances and will always be mixed into a carrier oil for use during a massage. A maximum of 3 per cent essential oil is all that is needed, that is 3 drops in a 5ml teaspoon of base oil. The base oil can be any natural vegetable oil. Grapeseed is popular as it is light, odourless and very easily absorbed by the skin, though almond and sunflower are often used to. Richer oils, such as wheatgerm, avocado, apricot kernel and jojoba, may be added in small quantities for drier skins or for use on the face. The aromatherapist will usually make up the oil just before each massage though he or she may also make up a larger quantity for the client to take home.

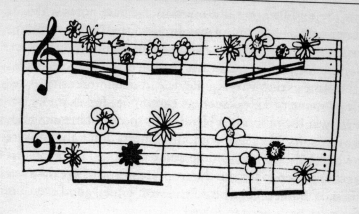

BLENDING ESSENTIAL OILS

On each visit, the aromatherapist will make up a blend of essential oils especially suited to you at that particular time. They will be chosen for their therapeutic powers and their effects upon the nervous system, but whichever oils are chosen they must produce a harmonious aroma. However good a blend may seem from a therapeutic viewpoint, if it smells awful, it certainly won't be of much use! Just as an individual oil is more powerful than the sum of its constituents, so a blend can be more powerful than each essential oil on its own. The various oils will often subtly enhance each other in some way.

An aromatherapist will know through experience which oils work well together and which don't and will usually have favourite blends. That does not mean that he or she won't sometimes make mistakes! The possible combinations are limitless, leaving plenty of scope for experimentation. There are, however, certain theories about blending oils which are said to lead to a harmonious blend.

Firstly, there is blending according to notes. As in classic perfumery, essential oils are divided into groups of top notes, middle notes and base notes. Top notes are the one we smell first in a blend and are the lightest and most volatile oils. Next come the middle notes, followed by the base notes which are heavier with a lingering aroma. In classic perfumery a mixture containing a top, middle and base note will produce a well balanced blend. The quantities of each oil will not necessarily be the same as they vary a great deal in odour intensity. A very little amount of an oil such as camomile, for example, will overpower the others in a blend. This theory of blending does have its faults. To begin with, the experts don't always agree on which oils are top, middle and base notes. Some oils will also change depending on the crop, season or where they were produced. Sometimes a blend still won't smell good even after these rules have been followed.

Blending by families is another way of mixing oils. These may either be botanical families or groups of oils from just trees or just herbs or just citrus fruits for example. Mixing oils from the same type or family of plants usually produces a pleasant blend. Sometimes combining families, such as citrus with spices, will work well. Some aromatherapists see oils in terms of colours. For example, an odour such as petitgrain (orange leaves) is green and fresh, whereas some marjorams are brown and earthy. Blending the colours may produce a harmonious blend. Indeed some therapists use colour healing, so the 'colour' of the oil will also have a therapeutic effect as well as the odour and chemical properties.

When the aromatherapist has mixed the blend, he or she will ask the client if they like it. The treatment won't be much good if the client finds the odour offensive. Sometimes the client will be asked which oil they prefer from a few different ones. There is a lot to be said for intuitive knowledge of what the body needs. The whole area of smell is highly subjective, but the experienced aromatherapisat will be able to select a blend that is of therapeutic value and also has an aroma to suit each client.

4
THINKING ABOUT AROMATHERAPY

Who goes to an aromatherapist? What do they do? How many sessions will I need? How do I find one? All these are questions people ask when thinking about aromatherapy, and in this chapter I'll attempt to answer these and others which might crop up.

Who goes to an aromatherapist?
Anyone and everyone, from babies to people in their nineties, can benefit. It is never too early or late to start aromatherapy. It is often a therapy which seems to appeal more to women than men, but both can benefit equally. You won't necessarily come out of the treatment room smelling like a perfume counter – aromas vary from the delicate floral types to the woody more 'masculine' smells.

What does an aromatherapist treat?
Medically qualified aromatherapists may choose to use essential oils to treat any condition, including serious life-threatening conditions such as infectious diseases or even AIDS. However, the majority of aromatherapists have clients with problems of a less serious nature. Some of the conditions which respond well to aromatherapy include nervous complaints such as stress, anxiety, depression and tension – both mental and physical; skin problems including eczema and acne and menstrual problems including pre-menstrual tension. Rheumatism and arthritis sufferers can feel great relief from

aromatherapy massage, usually combined with a change in diet. Circulatory disorders can be helped a great deal, as can respiratory problems. If your particular condition does not respond to the treatment, your aromatherapist will be able to refer you to another more suitable therapist – osteopath, homeopath, acupuncturist or other who may be able to help.

Essential oils can also be extremely effective in treating acute conditions, such as colds, sore throats, sinusitis, constipation, diarrhoea, headaches and migraine, conditions which are often treated at home by drugs bought over the counter at the chemist. With these drugs the symptoms clear up and the sufferer is happy until the condition recurs. In all these situations the problem is being suppressed without its real causes being investigated. Though it is not always possible to see the aromatherapist when a problem actually arises, by visiting your therapist regularly, he or she can talk to you about any recurring problems and help you to build up your own aromatherapy first aid kit to treat minor conditions as they occur (see Chapter 6).

Do I need to be ill to see an aromatherapist?
The answer to this is most definitely 'no'. Almost everyone will benefit from having a more relaxed mind and body. Aromatherapy is a wonderful preventative form of treatment. Circulation will be improved, it will help clear the body of toxins and increase the body's own potential to heal itself and fight off infection. Some people consider aromatherapy to be a luxurious treat, others feel it is an important part of their routine. Attitudes depend on whether we feel that having a well-balanced mind and body is something towards which we strive in order to weather the pressures of modern living or merely a pleasant interlude in a life normally full of stress and tension. Most of us lead a hectic life, whether we are dealing with vast sums of money on the stock exchange, coping with a home and young children, or these days perhaps both! It is important to stop once in a while and 'treat' ourselves to something that is just for us, something relaxing and nurturing. An aromatherapy session can provide that for everyone.

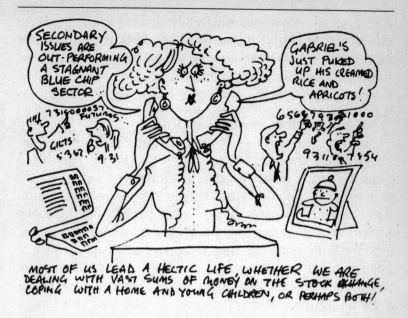

MOST OF US LEAD A HECTIC LIFE, WHETHER WE ARE DEALING WITH VAST SUMS OF MONEY ON THE STOCK EXCHANGE, COPING WITH A HOME AND YOUNG CHILDREN, OR PERHAPS BOTH!

Is there anyone who shouldn't see an aromatherapist?

Again the answer is 'no'. However, there are some medical conditions that your aromatherapist will need to know about which may affect his or her choice of oils and their method of application. These should come up in discussion at the initial consultation but just in case make sure your aromatherapist knows if you suffer from epilepsy, high blood pressure, if you have ever been treated for any form of cancer or if you are pregnant.

HOW DO I FIND A PRACTITIONER?

Aromatherapists work in a variety of places. Many have practices at home, others work in health clubs or sports centres. A local natural health clinic is often a good place to try. If they don't have an aromatherapist on the premises, they will often be able to recommend one who works locally. Beauty salons often advertise aromatherapy treatments where their therapists give a massage with ready blended oils. If this is the type of session you want then that's fine. However, if you want a personal consultation with a holistic practitioner than ask for further information before you book.

What qualifications should I look for?

There are many schools of aromatherapy around now, all giving their own diplomas. However, to be sure your aromatherapist has undergone a thorough training, check that the association to which they belong is a member of the Aromatherapy Organizations Council (AOC). The AOC has a core curriculum as a minimum standard for all its member organizations ensuring that their aromatherapists have a good grounding in the use of essential oils and massage, as well as anatomy and physiology. Most associations will have a list of qualified aromatherapists in your area (see Useful Addresses section on pages 110–112).

Making an appointment

In most cases you will need to book an appointment in advance. People either visit the practice or book by phone. Most centres have receptionists who will book the appointment and may ask you about the nature of your complaint. If they do, just give a very brief description so the practitioner will know what to expect. If you do have to cancel an appointment for some reason, you may be asked to give notice, usually 24 hours, otherwise you may have to pay a cancellation fee.

If your aromatherapist works from home they will probably have an answer phone. Do leave a message, they really will get back to you!

How long will a session take?

This does vary between therapists, depending on how and where they work. In general the first session will be longer, usually 1½ hours, though sometimes it could be two. Subsequent sessions are usually an hour in length, though again this could vary depending on the practitioner and the nature of the complaint.

How often will I need to go?

Again this will depend on your own particular needs and the way your chosen therapist works. Though you are likely to feel good after one session, like any alternative therapy it is not an instant cure. In cases where the complaint has taken months or years to develop, it may take some time before any improvement is seen. Other cases may respond very quickly but regular visits to the aromatherapist will have great preventative value. Many people think of an aromatherapy session as a treat. While this may be true, living as we do in a highly stressful and hectic environment, it is important to allow ourselves time for something beneficial and nurturing on a regular basis. A regular aromatherapy session, be it weekly or monthly, can help us to keep our balance and prevent illness from occurring.

How much does a session cost?

Charges vary from place to place, but the average in Britain is around £20 to £40. Some practitioners may charge more for the longer initial session. Oils for home use are usually included in the cost of the treatment.

When should I book a first appointment?

Obviously it will be better if you haven't eaten a large meal just before the visit as this could cause discomfort during the massage. Similarly it would be unwise to come to a session after drinking alcohol. It is often a good idea to allow yourself some time to relax before and after a session, especially on the first visit. Arriving hot and flustered can make it difficult for you to relax very quickly or dashing back to work straight away will soon make you forget how you felt during the session. Perhaps try booking your first appointment in the late afternoon so you can go home and relax afterwards. Remember if you are returning to work the chances are your hair will be a little oily and any make-up will have been removed so you may not want to attend any important meetings! If you're at home with children, try a session in the morning then allow yourself a bit of time to relax before they come home from school. On subsequent visits, when you know what to expect, you will probably be able to relax more easily at first and carry the benefits away with you in a calm manner.

Can I drive home afterwards?

It may seem like a silly question, but it is a good idea to tell the aromatherapist how you intend to get home. Some oils are extremely sedating and may impair your judgement for driving. You may be given some oils to take home for use later.

Do I have to take all my clothes off

As essential oils are applied on the skin for absorption then you will need to take some clothes off. For a full massage you will usually be asked to take off everything, or if you prefer you can leave your pants on. You will be given a large towel and during the massage the therapist will keep covered the parts of the body he or she isn't working on. If, however, you feel uncomfortable taking off all your clothes, then do tell the aromatherapist. One of the main aims is to create an atmosphere in which you can relax and feel comfortable. If at first this means you keep some clothes on then the aroma-therapist will work on what parts of the body he or she can, until you feel happy about removing the rest of your clothes.

Bearing in mind that you will have to take most of your clothes off for the massage, it is a good idea not to wear lots of fiddly garments which take a long time to take off and put back on. This includes jewellery as you will be asked to remove this as well.

How should I prepare for the visit?

On the first visit the aromatherapist will take a full case history (see Chapter 5). It will be helpful for the therapist and easier for you if you spend a few minutes beforehand thinking about

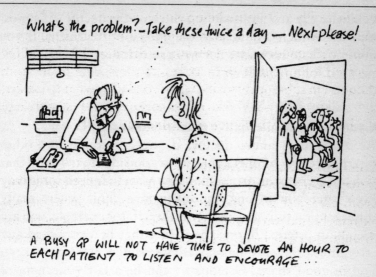

What's the problem? — Take these twice a day — Next please!

A BUSY GP WILL NOT HAVE TIME TO DEVOTE AN HOUR TO EACH PATIENT TO LISTEN AND ENCOURAGE...

some of the things you might be asked. These will include your past medical history and that of your family, your present lifestyle and the particular reason for your visit. Be prepared to answer questions about your mental and emotional state as well. The aromatherapist isn't being nosey but needs to know all about you before making the choice of oils.

Should I tell my doctor?

If you are seeing a doctor for any particular complaint or if you are taking a course of prescribed drugs then it is a good idea to tell him or her that you are planning to see an aromatherapist. The reaction may vary a great deal from highly sceptical to positively encouraging. However, whatever their opinion of essential oils, most doctors do recognize the benefits of regular massage. There is sometimes a great deal of antagonism between orthodox and alternative healthcare practitioners and we can do a lot to relieve this by actually talking to each other and complementing each other's skills. A busy general practitioner will not have time to devote an hour to each patient to listen and encourage them, so may be only too pleased to have someone else do this.

Likewise the aromatherapist will value the doctor's diagnostic skills which will help in the choice of treatment. If you communicate between your two practitioners there should be no need for any problems.

Can I see other alternative practitioners as well?

As with your family doctor, if you are seeing any other alternative practitioners, then it is a good idea to tell them that you are going to an aromatherapist as well. Indeed some may even refer you to one, especially in a clinic where many different practitioners work together. If, for example, you are seeing an osteopath, once he is sure that he's corrected any structural problems, he may advise regular massage to keep you in good shape. Osteopathy can be a fairly mechanical process, seeing an aromatherapist may help with the emotional side of the problem. Or perhaps you are seeing a homeopath or herbalist. These therapies will deal with both physical and emotional problems but don't involve any body contact, so again massage could fill in this side of things. If you are seeing a homeopath, it is especially important to tell him or her before you see the aromatherapist, as some essential oils may antidote the homeopathic remedies. Your homeopath may be able to write a note for the aromatherapist so that he or she knows which oils to avoid.

On the other hand, an aromatherapist may recommend that you see another alternative practitioner as well. If your back problem, for example, has not improved after a few sessions then the aromatherapist may ask you to see an osteopath for a second opinion. Or if the massage and essential oils bring up a lot of emotional problems or confusions, then some form of psychotherapy could be of great value. The main concern of any healthcare practitioner is your well-being, so they will work together however they can to find the best treatment for you.

5
THE FIRST VISIT

Having decided to have your first aromatherapy session, you might feel a little apprehensive when you arrive at the clinic or practitioner's home. Don't worry. Everything will be done to make you feel at ease. Most centres will have a receptionist who will explain the procedure and probably give you some information to read while you wait. The treatment rooms are clean and fresh looking, without the clinical appearance of many doctors' surgeries or dentists' waiting rooms. If the aromatherapist works from home, he or she will probably take you straight to the treatment room which will be furnished in soft relaxing colours. The main focus of the room will be the massage couch. Then there will be all the bottles of essential oils, base oils, creams and dishes and a pile of soft towels. This is of course a generalization, but there will be a genuine attempt to make you feel relaxed.

After taking off your coat, you will be asked to sit down, ready for the case history. The therapist may have a desk but often a couple of chairs are used to create a less formal atmosphere.

THE CASE HISTORY

The initial case history is an important part of your aromatherapy treatment. It will give the therapist details of your present condition and your lifestyle in general so he or she can choose a blend of oils especially for you.

To begin with you will be told a bit about aromatherapy and how the therapist works as an individual and also exactly what he or she will do during the session. Then your therapist will start your case history. Some aromatherapists will use printed sheets, others just a note pad. Don't be put off by this note taking, the aromatherapist needs to keep a detailed record for future use. After asking basic facts like name, address, date of birth, family status and occupation he or she will ask about the reason for the visit. This could be for a specific complaint or for relaxation or perhaps just curiosity.

If you have come about a specific condition then the aromatherapist will want to know as much as possible about it. You will be asked when it started and if anything else significant happened in your life at the same time. The aromatherapist will want to know what makes the condition better and what makes it worse. On a physical level, you will be asked to try to describe any pain or other symptoms, while on an emotional level you will be asked how you cope with the condition or even how your family cope with it. It is useful to have thought about some of these things beforehand. It is not easy to put such things as pain into words, but it will help the therapist greatly.

Previous medical history
As well as your present state of health, the aromatherapist will need to know about your past medical history. This will help in working out any underlying causes of a present condition and will also point out essential oils which should be avoided or any contra-indications to massage. For example, a recent operation or accident may mean modifying the massage to account for this. Or if you have ever suffered from epilepsy, then certain essential oils must be avoided. It is important for the aromatherapist to know about illnesses such as allergies, diabetes or heart conditions. You will also be asked about the medical history of members of your family, as there may be a predisposition toward certain illnesses which runs within the family. The aromatherapist will also want to know of any medication you have been prescribed in the past or are taking at present. Most women forget to mention the contraceptive pill, but it can be important to know.

Your body

Returning to the present, the aromatherapist will enquire about the vital functions of the body such as the digestive, respiratory and menstrual systems. You will be asked about any problems to do with digestion or bowel movements and perhaps about your appetite. The therapist will then move on to respiration – do you ever have problems breathing or suffer from catarrh or sinusitis? Women will be asked about their menstrual cycle – is it regular, do you get a lot of pain, do you suffer from premenstrual tension or are you going through the menopause? Moving on you will be asked about your circulation – do you often get cold hands or feet, do you know what your blood pressure is?

Having gathered lots of information on your basic bodily functions, the aromatherapist will ask about your general constitution. You will be asked if you get headaches frequently or catch colds more often than most people? Don't be afraid to mention any minor problem you may have at this point. It may seem unrelated but could nevertheless have some bearing on your general well-being.

You will also be asked about your sleeping pattern. Do you ever have any problems sleeping and if so how do they affect you? Perhaps you find it hard to get to sleep, or maybe you wake up in the middle of the night and can't sleep again. Some people feel they're getting enough sleep yet still wake up tired next morning. All this information will be useful when the aromatherapist chooses a suitable course of treatment.

Stress factors

The case history will now turn to more general questions about your lifestyle and the particular pressures you are under.

For many people a major area of stress stems from the workplace. So many jobs these days force us to work long hours in a less than ideal environment. We often think of stress at work being associated with the high-powered business executive, jet-setting around the world, but every job has its particular pressures. What about a nurse on night shifts

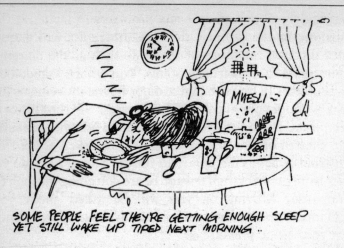

SOME PEOPLE FEEL THEY'RE GETTING ENOUGH SLEEP
YET STILL WAKE UP TIRED NEXT MORNING ..

in an understaffed ward or a housing officer in an inner city area? The actual working environment itself can be very stressful – a busy, smoky office with little natural light and full of VDU screens is a good example. How you actually spend your working day is also important – are you on your feet from nine till five, or are you sitting at a desk which is the wrong height for you? Or perhaps the problem is unemployment and all the pressures, both financial and emotional that this can bring. Don't immediately rule out aromatherapy because you can't afford it, ring up the aromatherapist as he or she may be able to offer you a concessionary rate.

For some people, however, stresses stem from home life not the workplace. Being a single parent, running a house as well as having a full-time job can put a lot of additional pressure on us or perhaps you are having problems with teenage children or financial difficulties. Your aromatherapist isn't going to pry into your personal life for the sake of it, but if there is something which is affecting either your physical or your emotional state then it is worth mentioning.

Diet and fitness

Our level of fitness will depend on many factors and can have a direct bearing on our well-being. Someone with a sedentary job who takes no form of exercise could run the risk of suffering from obesity or heart problems in later life. The active sportsman on the other hand brings the problems of sports injuries, from torn muscles to injured joints.

The foods we eat often have a direct bearing on our general health, but with some conditions, such as acne and arthritis, our diet is of vital importance in treating the condition. In such cases, the aromatherapist will need to know as much as possible about what you eat and will either offer dietary advice or perhaps refer you to a nutritionist. If you have no specific health complaint, then he or she will just enquire about your awareness of the right foodstuffs to eat and offer advice where appropriate (see Chapter 6).

When we are feeling under pressure many of us reach for some sort of stimulant, be it caffeine, nicotine or alcohol. We may get the lift we need for a short time but the effects soon wear off and we reach again for the coffee jar or cigarette packet. The aromatherapist is likely to ask you how much coffee, tea or alcohol you drink, whether or not you smoke, or if you use any form of drugs. Be honest! The aromatherapist needs to know, and although you will be offered advice, any decision to change these habits will be yours.

Your mind

Finally, the aromatherapist will ask you if there are any emotional problems you wish to talk about. For some people this is just the opportunity they need to talk to someone not involved in their life about a particular difficulty they are having. Sometimes just airing a problem gives you a clearer view to sorting it out. The right essential oils, with their powerful effect on the emotions, may put you in the right frame of mind to do this. On the other hand, if you don't feel comfortable about talking to a 'stranger' on such a personal level then you won't be forced into doing so. Once you've been for several sessions and have built up a relationship with your aromatherapist, then you will be able to talk about emotional matters if you need to.

Body language

In addition to asking lots of questions, the aromatherapist

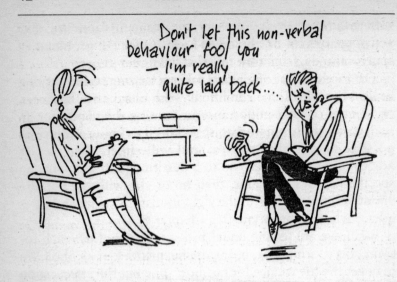

will be picking up lots of non-verbal clues. Body language can give away a lot about your personality, are you sitting in a comfortable relaxed way or are your shoulders hunched and fists clenched in a tense anxious manner? Do you arrive punctually, looking calm and collected or do you arrive hot and flustered, ten minutes late. Your general appearance can give plenty of information too, as can your complexion and posture. Don't worry about all these clues you are giving away, they too will help the aromatherapist build up a complete picture of you. He or she will then be able to make a choice of essential oils to suit your needs. Some aromatherapists, however, may use other techniques to either find out more information about you or to check the choice of oils.

THE BLEND OF OILS

Having taken a case history and used any diagnostic techniques necessary, the aromatherapist will be able to choose a mixture of oils for you. This will depend on many factors, from physical needs to your emotional state. It may also depend on what you are doing for the rest of the day. If you come before work, then a highly sedating blend would be inappropriate; similarly, stimulating oils would not be a good idea in the evening. If necessary, the aromatherapist will give you some oils to take home and use at night time. You may also be asked to smell the oils that have been chosen before a blend is mixed, or even asked which oils you prefer out of a small selection. If you don't like the blend that has been chosen, you won't enjoy having it massaged into you for an hour! We are also often far more intuitive than we think and are able to pick the oils that our bodies actually need.

THE MASSAGE

The next stage of the session is the massage. At this point you will be given a towel and asked to undress. The aromatherapist may leave the room but more likely he or she will be busy preparing the couch and mixing up your oils. Don't be embarrassed about taking your clothes off – the aromatherapist is quite used to seeing other people's bodies. When you are ready, you will be asked to lie on the couch, where the therapist will cover you with a towel and ask you if you feel comfortable. Don't be afraid to say if you are in any discomfort at any stage during the massage. Some people need support under their backs, others under their knees, if they lie on their back for any length of time.

As the massage begins, the aromatherapist will be looking for any clues as to the state of the muscles. Skin tone, swollen or raised areas, heat or cold can all give clues as to which areas need attention. While working, the aromatherapist will begin to get to know your body and its areas of tension. The best state in which to receive a massage is one of deep relaxation while still retaining an awareness of how the touch of the therapist feels. This is best achieved in silence. For many people this is a relief from the hustle and bustle of the day, but for some, this silence seems uncomfortable at first. Most of us aren't used to being in the company of just one other person without making any form of verbal communication. If this really is a problem the aromatherapist may play some soothing music or perhaps go through some relaxation exercise with you (see Chapter 6).

As described previously, the massage given by the aromatherapist will vary according to your particular needs – slow and soothing for relaxation, brisker if a more invigorating massage is needed. Particular attention will be paid to those parts of the body that need it most. For many people it is their shoulders or lower back, for others it could be work on their sinus points. Being relaxed but aware during a massage can throw up some surprising facts about ourselves. People with very ticklish feet are often amazed when they suddenly find the aromatherapist working on their foot without them dissolving into laughter. Other people find some areas far more sensitive than they imagined. If for some reason it doesn't feel quite right to be touched for example on your stomach, feet or perhaps even knees, then tell the aromatherapist and he or she will leave that area until you feel more comfortable. Massage can be an incredibly powerful therapy. When we hold in our emotions we tense various muscles, locking these emotions in. As the muscles are worked and begin to relax, some people feel these emotions being released. Don't worry if you feel like crying or get angry during a massage, it may be just what you need to do.

OTHER TECHNIQUES USED BY AROMATHERAPISTS

When working on particular clients some aromatherapists incorporate techniques from other therapies. Below are a few that may be used.

Reflexology

Reflexology or zone therapy has its origins in the ancient Eastern civilizations. The theory behind it is that there are reflexes located in the feet which correspond to every gland, organ and part of the body. If for some reason there is any disorder or blockage in energy flow in some part of the body, then crystalline deposits will be found at the corresponding reflex point on the foot. By feeling for these deposits on the foot the therapist will pick up on problem areas in the body often before the patient knows they exist. This can be a useful diagnostic tool for the aromatherapist, and may help in the choice of oils. Some aromatherapists are also qualified in reflexology, though it is probably unlikely that a therapist will do a full reflexology treatment along with the aromatherapy. Working on troubled reflexes can help rebalance the bodily systems, though it can be quite painful for the first time. Your aromatherapist is most likely to just press the reflex joints briefly to check for possible disorders and then begin an aromatherapy massage based on any information uncovered. If appropriate, a separate session concentrating only on reflexology may be suggested.

Touch for health

Applied kinesiology or touch for health, is a system based on the Eastern theory of energy lines or meridians and Western chiropractic knowledge. The theory is that there is a functional connection between specific muscle groups in the body and the energy pathways represented by acupuncture meridians. By testing the strength and tune of various muscle groups, the practitioner is able to detect any imbalances in the energy flow. The meridians correspond to the various organs in the body, such as the heart, bladder, kidneys etc. Touch for health practitioners believe that muscular weakness may be apparent prior to the symptoms of any disorder occurring. So as with reflexology, the therapist is able to detect disease before the patient is actually aware of any symptoms. As before, the aromatherapist may just use touch for health techniques as a diagnostic tool, or may actually work on appropriate points to correct any imbalances.

Touch for health has also proved very useful in detecting food allergies. When the client is exposed to a particular foodstuff to which they have an allergy, a muscle which was previously tested strong will become weak. Some aromatherapists use a similar test with essential oils. Their client holds a bottle of essential oil and a muscle test is performed. If the test is weak, then this oil is not suitable for that person, whereas if it is strong then the body will benefit from its use.

Dowsing

Another method used by some aromatherapists for checking their choice of oils is dowsing. This involves holding a small pendulum over the bottle of oil and asking certain questions, such as 'Is this oil right for this person?' The aromatherapist will then read the movements of the pendulum, which is usually clockwise for yes and anti-clockwise for no. Not all aromatherapists believe in the use of the pendulum in this way, but some do feel it makes a useful check once they have used other information to make a blend.

Shiatsu

Shiatsu is a Japanese style of massage, using finger pressure and the same system of meridians or energy lines as acupuncture. Shiatsu practitioners have undergone a thorough training and study of Oriental philosophies, but some aromatherapists know about the meridians and pressure points and pay attention to them during the massage. Shiatsu is not a smooth flowing massage in the same way that aromatherapy massage is, and is usually performed fully clothed. Some of the principles, however, can be applied and it can be particularly useful for helping the flow of energy or for drawing attention to an area of the body where the energy is blocked.

The chakras

The idea of the chakras comes from the Eastern philosophy of tantric yoga. They are seven energy centres spaced up the spine from its base to the top of the head. Each is associated with a gland, certain bodily systems, various mental aspects or emotions and one or more colours. The throat chakra, for example, is associated with the thyroid gland, the respiratory system and alimentary canal are seen as its creative centre and its corresponding colours are blue and green. Some aromatherapists will tune into these centres while they work to see if they can detect any energy blocks. This can also be done with a pendulum, as with dowsing for the right essential oil (see page 46). Balancing the energy in the chakras is said to revitalize the body and develop self awareness.

Colour healing

Colour healing dates back to ancient Egypt and is closely connected with the ideas of the chakras (see above). We are attracted to certain colours because they have the same vibrational energy as our auras and are repelled by other colours because of a difference in wavelength. Colour therapists believe that by 'transmitting' appropriate colours via the chakras, they can balance the body, mind and spirit. On a less esoteric level, colour is known to have an effect on our mood and emotions. This is shown in our choice of colours for clothes or the colours we decorate a room with. Indeed, you are unlikely to find an aromatherapist's room decorated in harsh primary colours. Pastel colours, healing greens, calming yellows or warming pinks are much more likely to have been used.

Spritual healing

Spiritual healing has existed for thousands of years in all cultures and takes two forms – laying on of hands and distant healing where the healing is performed in the absence of the patient. It is the former that some aromatherapists use while working. Like other holistic practitioners, spiritual healers hold the belief that disease is the result of disharmony from within. They seek to restore balance throughout the whole person including physical, mental and spiritual aspects. Healers see themselves as a link between human life and some greater life force and act as channels for energy to pass from one to the other. If an aromatherapist uses spiritual healing, he or she may or may not tell the client and it will be up to them whether or not they choose to receive this energy, on either a conscious or sub-conscious level.

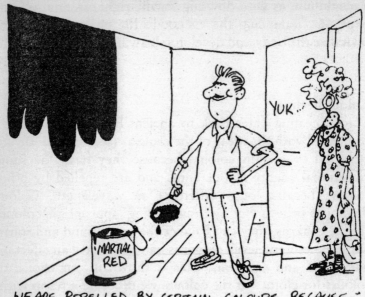

WE ARE REPELLED BY CERTAIN COLOURS BECAUSE THEY HAVE A DIFFERENT VIBRATIONAL ENERGY FROM OUR AURAS...

THE END OF THE SESSION

Whatever techniques the aromatherapist has used, the massage has to come to an end. After finishing the massage the aromatherapist will tell you to relax quietly on the couch for a few minutes. He or she may leave the room to allow you to do this in peace. When you feel ready to move, do so slowly, wriggle your toes and fingers, take some deep breaths and finally have a gentle stretch. If you have been in a state of deep relaxation, you will need time to come back down to earth. When you are ready, you can get off the couch and begin to get dressed.

At this point the aromatherapist will talk to you about further sessions. If there is a particular complaint that needs treating, then you may be asked to come on a weekly basis for the next few weeks. Otherwise it will be up to you when you next visit. It is, however, a good idea to book your next session as you leave, as it is all too easy to let the weeks slip by without realizing it. Building regular aromatherapy sessions into your schedule is a very good way of keeping healthy and coping with the pressures of everyday life.

Payment for the session will usually be made at the reception desk in a clinic or health centre or directly to the therapist if he or she works at home. If you would like regular sessions but genuinely cannot afford it, then do ask about the possibility of a concessionary rate for a course of treatment.

The next chapter deals with ways of using aromatherapy at home between sessions and also other techniques to help cope with stress and aid relaxation.

6
AROMATHERAPY
AT HOME

GETTING STARTED

The first thing you will need to do is buy some aromatherapy products. You have two choices – either buy your products off the shelf or buy some essential oils and mix your own. Professional aromatherapists will always blend their own oils and are often quite scathing about ready made products. While you wouldn't expect an aromatherapist to use these products in a treatment session, I think they do have a place for home use provided they are well chosen.

Ready blended products

The cosmetic industry has discovered essential oils recently and now many high street stores have aromatherapy ranges. They do have the advantage of being convenient, easy to use, safe and will probably cost you less initially. The disadvantages are that you will have less scope for experimentation and that these products will not be suitable for all methods of application. You also need to beware of products that are labelled 'aromatherapy' but in fact contain very little essential oil or contain it in a way that will not be of great benefit to the body. Below are some guidelines for choosing ready made products.

- Buy oil-based products such as bath oils or massage oils or lotions. While aromatherapy shower gels or face washes will smell nice and be effective as cleansers, don't expect to gain much benefit from the essential oils as they will not be in contact with the skin for long enough.

- Look for products which list the ingredients – this way you will be able to see exactly what you are buying. If you are unsure about anything contained in the product ask for advice. Honest and knowledgeable sales staff are often a good indication of the quality of the products.
- Try and find out the dilution of essential oils in a product. Ideally it should be between 1 per cent and 5 per cent depending on the essential oils used.

Mixing your own oils

If you do become interested in aromatherapy then there is no substitute for buying a collection of pure essential oils and blending them yourself. However, the oils must be used with care as they are very concentrated, so follow the guidelines for dilution listed below and if you have any doubts ask your aromatherapist. Here is a list of things you will need to get started.

Essential oils – These are the most important elements of your home aromatherapy kit and also the most costly so choose wisely. Chapter 2 (pages 12–13) discusses purity of essential oils and finding a reputable stockist. Listed below is information about some of the most common and useful essential oils. Build up your collection gradually getting to know a few oils well and adding new ones as the need arises.

Carrier oils – The essential oils need to be mixed into a base oil before use in order to dilute them and to enable them to be applied easily to the body. You may be able to find a basic carrier such as grapeseed oil in a supermarket and chemists will usually sell sweet almond oil. Your essential oil stockist will normally sell any others and will often stock a blend of base oils suitable for the face, body or for use in the bath. Find information below on the properties of some common carrier oils.

Creams and lotions – You may wish to add essential oils to face moisturizers and body lotions. Again essential oil stockists may sell base products for this purpose. Alternatively buy an unfragranced product made from a high proportion of natural ingredients. You can also make your own but remember that these will be unpreserved so will only have a very short life and must be kept in the fridge.

Bottles and labels – Any oils that you make up should be stored in dark glass bottles. These are easily obtained from a chemists. It is best to make small quantities regularly and always label them with the contents and the date they were made. The bottles can be reused provided they are thoroughly washed, or sterilized if possible, and dried before refilling.

METHODS OF APPLICATION

Details of how essential oils are administered are given in Chapter 3, but here are some ideas of how to gain maximum benefit from home treatment and the dilutions suitable for each method of application. Some oils can cause irritation to sensitive skins so begin with half the normal dilution stated and increase if no reaction is experienced. The same applies when using oils for elderly people and children. A separate section for pregnant women and babies is included at the end of this chapter.

Baths

A long soak in an aromatherapy bath is an ideal way to benefit from essential oils at home. Run a deep bath of water that is comfortably warm but not too hot and add the aromatherapy oils just before you get in. Keeping the door and windows shut will keep the steam in so you benefit from the evaporated oils as well. If you are mixing your own essential oils it is always preferable to mix them into a carrier oil first to ensure they are well dissolved. The oil will sit on the surface of the water and coat the skin as you get out leaving it feeling smooth and soft.

Pat your self dry so as not to remove too much of the oil. If you really don't like the feel of oil in a bath then try to find a product which disperses in the water or add the essential oils directly to the bath making sure you swirl the water around well to spread the oil.

To make your own bath oils, mix 50ml of carrier oil with 50 drops of one or a blend of essential oils and store in a dark glass bottle. Add 1 or 2 teaspoons (5–10ml) to each bath. If you are adding the oils directly to the water use 4 to 8 drops.

Inhalations

This is an ideal way of using aromatherapy for any condition concerned with air passages, such as sore throats, blocked noses or coughs. The same process can also be used to steam the face. Half fill a glass or crockery kitchen bowl with near boiling water and add about 3 drops of one or more essential oils. Cover your head with a towel, close your eyes and breathe in (see page 20 for more details). You can also put a few drops of oil onto a handkerchief or inhale directly from the bottle when you are out or at night but be careful not to let the oils come into contact with your nose.

Vaporization

Fill your home with the fragrance of essential oils by using an oil burner (see page 22 for possibilities). Add 5 to 8 drops of essential oil to your source of heat and allow the oil to evaporate. Do not use any form of carrier oil for this method as it can get overheated and smell unpleasant.

Compresses

This method can be used when massage is not advised i.e. with sprains, or if you don't want to be touched or to take a bath as in the case sometimes with headaches. Add about 6 drops of essential oil to half a pint of either hot or cold water (see page 21). Put a flannel or a piece of lint on top of the water, wring out and apply to the affected area. Leave until the compress has returned to body temperature, then re-apply as above. Repeat three to six times until the pain has eased.

Massage

As we have already seen, massage is probably the best way of using essential oils yet it is the most difficult to manage for home use. You have two options, massage yourself or ask a friend to give you a massage. There are many excellent massage books on the market, so have a look around before you buy to find one which suits your needs (see Further Reading page 114 for some ideas). If you become really interested, many massage practitioners run workshops, sometimes through local education authorities so they are quite inexpensive.

Self-massage

Massaging yourself is not the same as being massaged by someone else, as you are the one doing all the work. Therefore it is not especially relaxing but it still has many positive benefits, including improving circulation, toning muscles and tissue and increasing self-awareness. Find a book with a self-massage sequence and follow this, but you can also be quite intuitive and listen to what your body needs. Only a few basic rules apply. One is in general to work towards the heart, that is up the legs and arms. Use long smooth strokes to begin with followed by more vigorous kneading movements once the muscles are warm. When massaging the stomach always go in a clockwise direction, following the path of the digestive system. Be gentle with the delicate skin of the face, especially around the eyes. The hardest part to massage, and unfortunately the part most often needing attention, is the back. Reach the top of your shoulders and knead well and try using your fists for the rest of your back. You can always try one of those long-handled massage rollers that are popular at the moment.

Do-in is the self-massage form of the Japanese massage, shiatsu (see page 46). It tends to be a fairly vigorous form of massage, which can be quite invigorating and energizing. If you are lucky you may be able to find a *do-in* class, otherwise some of the shiatsu books now on the market have sequences to follow.

Massaging others

A good way to receive massage at home is to learn together with a friend or partner. Find a good book and read it thoroughly before you start and take it in turns to give and receive a massage. It is probably better to start very simply, adding one new stroke at a time rather than trying to follow a whole sequence from the book while massaging. Also practise the strokes that your aromatherapist uses on you and ask your partner how they feel. So long as you avoid too deep pressure and don't work on the spine itself you won't do any harm. Make sure your partner feels warm and comfortable and try to tune into their needs. Warm the oil in your hands before you start and try to be conscious of your own posture as well. Begin by using long smooth strokes and as you get more confident try some different ones. Don't worry about getting it 'right': as long as it feels good to the receiver then it is fine. It can be a rewarding experience for you as well as a relaxing one for your partner and vice versa.

To make your own massage oil, add 30 drops of essential oil to 50ml of carrier oil and store in a dark glass bottle. Alternatively make up as required using 3 drops of essential oil to each teaspoon (5ml) of carrier oil.

THE ESSENTIAL OILS

The following list of essential oils is by no means exhaustive but it includes most of the commonly used ones and all those mentioned in the following sections of this book. The oils are listed alphabetically and are described under four headings:

aroma, price, properties and precautions which cover the following information:

Aroma – Gives a brief description of the fragrance, though as this is such a personal thing it is always a good idea to smell the oil before you buy.

Price – This gives an idea of the price band that each oil falls into. An aromatherapist will always choose the oils for their therapeutic qualities regardless of the price. It can, however, be a costly business building up a set of essential oils for home use and price can be an important factor in your choice. The price bands are:

- Cheap – under £5 per 10ml
- Medium – £5–£10 per 10ml
- Expensive – over £10 per 10ml

N.B. you may have to pay a higher price for organic oils.

Properties – This section covers the properties of each oil which are most relevant for the person wishing to use them for self-help at home.

Precautions – States whether the oil should be avoided by anyone such as epileptics or pregnant women, and if it should be used in a weaker dilution than usual.

Basil
Aroma – Fresh, sharp, almost aniseed like.
Price – Cheap.
Properties – An excellent oil for clearing the head and relieving headaches. It can also be helpful for promoting mental clarity, and in cases of insomnia when this is due to thoughts churning around in the mind. In this case always mix it with a more soporific oil such as lavender because basil on its own is quite stimulating. It can also be used for aching, overworked muscles.

Precautions – Do not use during pregnancy. Use in low dilution as it may irritate the skin.

Bergamot

Aroma – Fresh and citrus with floral notes.
Price – Medium.
Properties – A refreshing and uplifting oil, bergamot is an ideal 'pick-me-up' if you are feeling down or depressed. It is also useful to aid recovery from illness, especially if this has been caused by a virus. It is a good choice for oily skin and can be beneficial for treating acne because of its antiseptic action.
Precautions – Increases the skin's photosensitivity so avoid strong sunlight after use because it contains bergaptene. It is possible to buy it bergapteneless in which case the above precaution is not applicable.

Black pepper

Aroma – Sharp and spicy.
Price – Medium.
Properties – Black pepper increases local circulation so it is an excellent oil for warming the muscles prior to exercise and for easing aches and pains afterwards. It can also be used in conditions associated with sluggish circulation such as cellulite and fluid retention. One drop can be added to a blend to give it more warmth and spice.
Precautions – Use in low dilution as it may irritate the skin.

Camomile

Aroma – Sweet, fruity and lightly floral.
Price – Expensive.
Properties – There are many differnt types of camomile (sometimes seen as chamomile) though the one most suitable for home use is Roman camomile. You may also come across German camomile which is blue in colour and has a strong, less pleasing aroma. In all aspects of its action, camomile can be said to be calming and soothing. Because of its analgesic

properties, it works well on dull aches and pains whether it is backache, period pains or stomach ache. It is great for calming you down if you are feeling irritable or angry and can help promote a good night's sleep. It is excellent on any skin condition that is red and sore and can provide relief from itching. As a mild and gentle oil, it is the first choice for babies and children.

Precautions – Avoid during the first three months of pregnancy.

Cinnamon

Aroma – Warm, sweet and spicy.

Price – Cheap.

Properties – A very warming oil which can be used to ease muscular aches and pains and menstrual cramps. It can be used in the bath when you are feeling chilled and is wonderful used in an oil burner with citrus oils such as orange for a winter fragrance.

Precautions – Always buy cinnamon leaf oil as the bark produces an oil which is too irritating on the skin. Even cinnamon leaf is very powerful so use in low dilutions.

Clary sage

Aroma – Herbal, warm and nutty.

Price – Medium.

Properties – It is a warming and relaxing oil useful for headaches caused by chronic tension and for period pains. As it has an affinity with the uterus it can be used to bring on an overdue period and to aid contractions during labour. On a mental level its action is often described as euphoric though some people find that it makes them very drowsy. It can also be used to balance excessively oily skin.

Precautions – Do not use when pregnant. Avoid drinking alcohol when using clary sage as it can lead to a hangover. Some people find they feel too drowsy to drive after using this oil.

Eucalyptus
Aroma – Fresh, strong and piercing.
Price – Cheap.
Properties – Eucalyptus is probably best known for its action on the respiratory tract, making an excellent inhalation to clear a blocked nose or ease a cough or sore throat. As an anti-viral agent it is also useful for preventing colds. It can also help to cool the body in feverish conditions and can help ease muscular aches and pains.
Precautions – A powerful oil so use in low dilutions.

Fennel
Aroma – Very fresh, green and herbal.
Price – Cheap.
Properties – A cleansing oil which can help the body eliminate toxins making it a good choice for hangovers and cellulite. It is also useful for regulating periods because of its hormonal action. It is said to promote the flow of breast milk.
Precautions – Do not use during pregnancy or for anyone with epilepsy. Do not use over a prolonged period of time but alternate with other oils.

Frankincense
Aroma – Warm, sweet and resinous.
Price – Medium.
Properties – Frankincense is also sometimes known as olibanum and is a deeply relaxing oil. It is said to slow and deepen the breathing and is excellent for states of anxiety. Many people use it in a burner during meditation. On a physical level it works well on the lungs, easing the tightness felt with asthma and helping chesty coughs. It is ideal to use at night as it will promote deep sleep as well. It is also an excellent oil for dry and ageing skin as it has a toning effect if the skin is slack.
Precautions – None known.

Geranium
Aroma – Floral, sweet and slightly lemony.

Price – Medium.

Properties – The key word to describe geranium is balancing. It is one of the oils which is calming yet uplifting at the same time, and can help a person feel more centred or grounded. It has a regulating effect on the hormonal system and can be extremely useful for helping PMS, while its diuretic properties can help with water retention and cellulite. It is a lovely oil to use for skin care and is thought to balance sebum production so it is suitable for any skin type.

Precautions – Do not use during pregnancy.

Grapefruit

Aroma – Sweet, citrus.

Price – Cheap.

Properties – As you would imagine from its fragrance, grapefruit has uplifting and reviving properties. It can be useful to beat fatigue and is helpful during pregnancy for this reason and also to help ease puffiness in the legs and hands.

Precautions – Use in low dilutions and avoid strong sunlight after use.

Jasmine

Aroma – sweet, intensely floral and heavy.

Price – Expensive.

Properties – One of the best oils to use during childbirth, jasmine strengthens contractions and eases pain. It is also useful in states of depression especially where there is a lack of self-confidence. It makes a luxurious skin-care oil for dry skin.

Precautions – Do not use during pregnancy until the week before the due date. As the oil is so concentrated, low dilutions are usually adequate.

Juniper

Aroma – Fresh and clean with woody notes.

Price – Medium.

Properties – Juniper is a very cleansing and detoxifying oil, and conditions which benefit from these properties include cellulite, over-indulgence in alcohol or rich food and acne. It can also be mentally cleansing if you have been in contact with a lot of people, especially if you feel you have picked up other's bad vibes!

Precautions – Do not use during pregnancy.

Lavender

Aroma – Distinctive, clean and floral.

Price – Cheap.

Properties – You will see when looking through the following sections that lavender is probably the most versatile and widely used essential oil and is a must for any home aromatherapy kit. On a physical level its analgesic properties make it useful for muscular aches and pains, headaches and period pains. It is antiseptic and healing and it can be used neat on cuts and burns. It is a great oil for all skin types as it encourages the renewal of skin cells. It is said to have a balancing effect on the emotions and will help to promote a good night's sleep.

Precautions – Do not use during the first three months of pregnancy.

Lemon

Aroma – Fresh, sharp citrus.

Price – Cheap.

Properties – An ideal oil for the circulatory system, lemon can be used in a massage oil to prepare the muscles for physical activity. It is also very cleansing and can be used in blends to help with cellulite. It is very refreshing and makes a good morning bath oil in combination with others.

Precautions – Use in low dilutions as it could irritate sensitive skin.

Lime

Aroma – Fresh and slightly sweet citrus.

Price – Cheap.

Properties – A stimulating oil which is useful to ease the symptoms of a cold such as catarrh, coughs and sore throats.

It can also be used to cool feverish conditions and to restore energy after illness. On a mental level it can restore vitality when there is tiredness and apathy.

Precautions – Use in low dilutions and avoid strong sunlight after use.

Mandarin

Aroma – Clear, fresh and orangey.

Price – Cheap.

Properties – A cheerful and 'happy' oil which is often recommended during pregnancy and childhood. Mixed with neroli it can help prevent stretch marks and generally promote a feeling of well-being. It can calm the mind when feeling anxious.

Precautions – Avoid strong sunlight after use.

Marjoram

Aroma – Herbal, nutty and quite sharp.

Price – Medium.

Properties – A warming oil with analgesic properties, Marjoram is useful to ease aching muscles and painful periods. As it increases circulation locally it can be used for headaches and migraines which stem from tension in the back of the neck. It can have a warming effect on the emotions as well and is an excellent for promoting a good night's sleep.

Precautions – Do not use during pregnancy.

Neroli

Aroma – Light, green, fresh and floral.

Price – Expensive.

Properties – Neroli comes from the blossom of the orange tree and is an extremely calming oil for states of anxiety. It can be used the day before a big event to calm the nerves and ensure a good night's sleep. It can also help in cases of diarrhoea and other stomach upsets which are brought on by stress. As a skin-care oil it has the ability to promote cell regeneration

making it ideal for mature skin and for the prevention of stretch marks.
Precautions – None.

Orange
Aroma – Sweet, fruity and citrus.
Price – Cheap.
Properties – More relaxing than most citrus oils yet still with that uplifting quality. It is warming and comforting and can ease muscular aches and pains. It can also help with cases of insomnia especially if mixed with lavender or neroli. It seems to spread sunshine on gloomy thoughts and makes a great bath oil to use during winter.
Precautions – Use in low dilutions as it can irritate sensitive skin.

Peppermint
Aroma – Fresh, cooling and minty.
Price – Cheap.
Properties – The cool, fresh smell of peppermint is ideal for clearing the head when mental clarity is needed and to relieve tension headaches. It also makes a good addition to an inhalation to clear the sinuses and promote easier breathing. It is commonly used to aid digestion, though peppermint tea is probably best advised for home use. Sniffing a few drops on a hanky can help quell feelings of nausea, especially caused by travel sickness.
Precautions – Do not use during pregnancy or when breast-feeding as it may slow up the supply of breast milk. Use in low dilutions as it can cause skin irritation.

Petitgrain
Aroma – Green, slightly floral and woody.
Price – Cheap.
Properties – Petitgrain comes from the leaves of the bitter orange tree and its properties are therefore somewhat similar to that of neroli. It is calming on the emotions yet refreshing at the same time. It blends well with many other essential oils

and is an excellent choice for bath oils. Mixed with its two companions from the orange tree, neroli and orange, it makes a wonderfully rounded and balancing oil.

Precautions – None known.

Rose

Aroma – Sweet, warm and very floral.

Price – Expensive.

Properties – Rose is typically viewed as a feminine oil and it is useful for regulating the menstrual cycle and helping with PMS, especially if the woman feels weepy and irritable. In cases of depression it can help to raise the spirits and restore self-confidence and self-esteem. It is an excellent choice for skin care, particularly for dry or mature skin and for thread veins.

Precautions – Do not use during pregnancy.

Rosemary

Aroma – Very sharp, clean and herbal.

Price – Cheap.

Properties – A stimulating oil which is ideal for muscular aches and pains particularly of an acute nature. It can also be used to prepare the muscles before a sporting event. Its diuretic properties combined with its effect on the circulation make it useful for conditions such as cellulite. It also has a stimulating effect on the mind and makes a good addition to a blend of oils for a morning bath and for times when energy levels are low. It can also relieve period pain and bring on late periods.

Precautions – Do not use during pregnancy. Best avoided by epileptics and those suffering from high blood pressure.

Sandalwood

Aroma – Exotic, sweet and woody.

Price – Expensive.

Properties – An extremely relaxing oil which is ideal to promote a good night's sleep. As a pulmonary antiseptic, it is also useful for treating dry, chesty coughs especially if they are

persistent at night. Sandalwood also makes a wonderful oil for dry, ageing skin.
Precautions – None known.

Tea-tree
Aroma – Fresh, woody and slightly spicy.
Price – Cheap.
Properties – Tea-tree has been discovered relatively recently as an essential oil and is now widely used because of its antiseptic, anti-viral and fungicidal properties. It is ideal for fighting any form of infection, and has a dual action as it stimulates the body's immune system at the same time. It is invaluable for colds and flu and as a first-aid oil for cuts and spots.
Precautions – Use in low dilutions as it may irritate sensitive skin.

Ylang Ylang
Aroma – Very sweet, floral and heady.
Price – Medium.
Properties – This intensely floral oil is very calming and relaxing and can help to slow over-rapid breathing associated with panic or shock. As it has a balancing effect on sebum production it is suitable for any skin type.
Precautions – Prolonged use may cause headaches.

AROMATHERAPY FOR EVERYDAY AILMENTS

Aromatherapy is a holistic treatment which looks at the causes of illness rather than just the symptoms. There are times, however, when essential oils can be invaluable in helping relieve the symptoms of those everyday complaints when it would be all too easy to reach for the aspirin bottle. Listed below are some of the ailments which respond well to aromatherapy with the most appropriate oils to use. Where possible I have discussed the possible causes and suggested different essential oils for each. If your symptoms persist or recur it is always best to see an aromatherapist or other alternative practitioner or your GP.

For each of the conditions I have suggested several oils to choose from. Pick your favourites from your collection and use them singly or in a blend. By experimenting with different oils for each condition you will find which ones work best for you. When making your own blends use the dilutions listed above and read the information on each oil to check for any possible contraindications or precautions. Alternatively I have suggested some blends for you to try. The recipes make a small bottle of oil, enough for several applications. Use 1 or 2 teaspoonfuls in the bath or as much as necessary for a massage.

Aches and pains
Whether through too much digging in the garden or day after day sitting at a computer, your muscles often come in for a hammering resulting in stiffness and soreness. A soak in an aromatherapy bath can work wonders, as can massaging the muscles to help ease away any knots. Never use massage if you have torn a muscle or sprained a ligament.

Prevention is better than cure
Athletes always warm up before an event to prevent muscle damage or soreness. Essential oils massaged in or used in a bath before any form of physical exercise can really help this process. Oils to use include:
- Rosemary
- Black Pepper
- Juniper

Sports rub – I massaged the following blend into the legs of two runners during their training period and prior to running a half marathon. Both reported no muscle stiffness after the race.

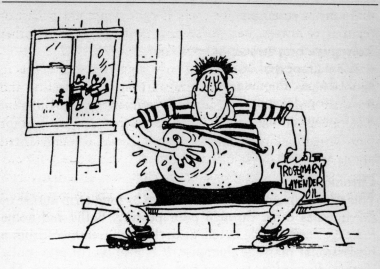

- 50 ml almond or grapeseed oil
- 20 drops rosemary
- 5 drops black pepper
- 5 drops orange

Pre-sports bath oil
- 50ml grapeseed oil
- 20 drops juniper
- 20 drops rosemary
- 10 drops lemon

Overworked muscles
Relieve the stiffness and soreness caused by over exertion by using:
- Rosemary
- Lavender
- Camomile
- Orange

Post work-out massage or bath oil – Good for aching legs and arms.
- 50ml almond or grapeseed oil
- 15 drops lavender

- 15 drops rosemary

Aching back bath soak
- 50ml grapeseed oil
- 20 drops camomile
- 20 drops lavender
- 10 drops orange

Chronic tension

This type of muscular ache is built up by long-term misuse of the muscles often through poor posture. Baths and home massage can provide excellent back up to treatment from a professional massage therapist. It is also worth preventing further discomfort by trying to correct your posture. The Alexander Technique is a way of becoming more aware of balance, posture and movement in everyday activities. Also ensure that you are provided with the correct equipment if the problem is work related. Essential oils to use at home include:
- Lavender
- Marjoram
- Camomile
- Clary sage
- Cinnamon

Warming shoulder and back rub
- 50ml almond or grapeseed oil
- 15 drops lavender
- 10 drops marjoram
- 5 drops cinnamon

Relaxing bath oil – Use before bed to ease away tension in the muscles and ensure a good night's sleep.
- 50ml grapeseed oil
- 20 drops clary sage
- 20 drops lavender
- 5 drops cinnamon
- 5 drops orange

Colds and influenza

These days the distinction between a bad cold and 'flu is somewhat confused. I know some people who suffer from 'flu several times a year while others who appear equally unwell only ever get colds! True influenza is a serious and debilitating infection which often occurs in epidemics and leads to secondary infections such as bronchitis if not treated. It goes without saying that a doctor should always be consulted if this is the case, especially if the sufferer is a child or elderly person. Essential oils can be used as a back up at home in addition to any more orthodox treatment. The suggestions below deal with the less serious conditions of colds and 'flu.

Preventative measures

If you can detect a cold at the very early stages you can sometimes prevent it developing further, or can lessen the severity if it does develop. Oils to use are:

- Tea-tree
- Eucalyptus
- Lavender

'Nip it in the bud' bath oil – Have some of this oil made up ready and jump into the bath the minute you feel the cold coming on. Try to go straight to bed afterwards and have two or three more baths over the next few days.

- 50ml grapeseed oil
- 30 drops lavender
- 20 drops tea-tree

Oil burner blend – Fill the top of an essential oil burner with water and add:

- 5 drops eucalyptus
- 5 drops lavender

Easing the symptoms of a cold

If you don't manage to prevent the cold from developing then essential oils can be used to help ease the symptoms and speed up recovery. Plenty of rest is advised as is a light wholefood diet, ideally consisting of lots of raw fruit and vegetables and fluids such as water and herbal teas. A combination of peppermint, elderflower and yarrow is a good blend of herbs for fighting a cold. The essential oils and blends listed above are also useful once the cold has developed with some additional ones for some of the more specific complaints. The full list includes:

- Tea-tree
- Lavender
- Eucalyptus
- Peppermint
- Bergamot
- Rosemary
- Marjoram

An inhalation for a blocked nose – To a bowl of near boiling water add:

- 2 drops eucalyptus
- 2 drops peppermint
- 2 drops tea-tree

This blend is very stimulating and therefore is best used during the day. For a night-time inhalation use:

- 4 drops lavender
- 2 drops eucalyptus *or* peppermint *or* tea-tree

A night-time bath to aid sleep and ease aches and pains

- 50ml grapeseed oil
- 20 drops lavender
- 20 drops marjoram
- 10 drops bergamot

A blend to aid recovery – Use the following for a morning bath which will help as a general tonic and help to restore energy levels once the cold is coming to an end.

- 50ml grapeseed oil
- 20 drops bergamot
- 20 drops rosemary
- 10 drops lime

Coughs and sore throats

A cough can persist long after a cold has cleared up and it is always worth consulting an alternative practitioner or your GP if these self-help measures are not effective after a few days of use. Effective oils are:

- Lavender
- Eucalyptus
- Sandalwood
- Frankincense

An inhalation for a tickly cough and sore throat – For daytime use, add to a bowl of near boiling water:

- 5 drops eucalyptus
- 5 drops lavender

For night-time use, add to a bowl of near boiling water:

- 5 drops lavender
- 5 drops sandalwood

Breathe through the mouth for maximum effect.

A massage oil for a chesty cough – Apply this blend to the chest and upper back especially at night-time to ease the cough and promote sleep.

- 50ml almond oil
- 10 drops frankinscense
- 10 drops lavender
- 10 drops sandalwood

Headaches

Headaches have many causes – sitting too long at a computer screen, tension in the neck or too much alcohol! Knowing what triggers your headaches may help you to prevent them and can help you choose the most appropriate aromatherapy treatment. If you regularly suffer from headaches which don't appear to have an obvious cause it may be worth consulting an alternative practitioner who may be able to shed some light on the matter. Migraine sufferers in particular often trace their headaches to particular foodstuffs.

Headaches caused by environmental factors

These headaches are often felt across the forehead and temples and can be caused by fluorescent lighting, over-crowded places or too much noise. Pain-relieving oils are needed and some of the most effective are:

- Lavender
- Basil
- Peppermint

A *head-clearing blend* – If you can bear to touch your head, massage this blend into your forehead, concentrating on temples and also across the scalp. Alternatively add it to a warm bath.

- 50ml grapeseed oil
- 20 drops lavender
- 5 drops basil
- 5 drops peppermint

A *cold compress* – Fill a bowl with cold water and add:

- 5 drops lavender
- 5 drops peppermint

Soak a flannel in the water, wring out and place across the forehead. Repeat as necessary.

Tension headaches

Tight muscles in the neck can restrict the small blood capillaries there resulting in throbbing headaches and some-times migraines. Oils which can help are:

- Marjoram
- Rosemary
- Clary sage
- Lavender

A *neck and shoulder rub for tension headaches* – Apply this oil to the back of the neck, across the shoulders and into the scalp or use in the bath.

- 50ml grapeseed oil
- 20 drops lavender
- 20 drops marjoram
- 10 drops rosemary

A hot compress – Fill a bowl with hand-hot water and add:
- 5 drops marjoram
- 3 drops clary sage
- 2 drops lavender

Soak a flannel in the water, wring out and place across the neck. Repeat as necessary.

Hangovers
Over-indulgence in alcohol, while best avoided, is something we all do on occasions. The best cures centre around helping the body eliminate the accumulated toxins and include drinking lots of water, taking a vitamin C supplement and doing some gentle exercise. Essential oils which help are:
- Juniper
- Lemon
- Fennel
- Rosemary
- Geranium

A morning-after bath
- 50ml grapeseed oil
- 20 drops juniper
- 10 drops fennel
- 10 drops lemon

An invigorating body oil – Take a warm shower then, if you can stand it, a quick cold one. Massage in the following blend while the skin is still damp.
- 50ml almond or grapeseed oil
- 15 drops geranium
- 10 drops rosemary
- 5 drops juniper

Minor injuries

Essential oils can form part of an everyday first-aid kit along with herbal and homeopathic remedies. Oils to include are:

- Lavender
- Tea-tree
- Camomile
- Fennel

Bruises

Probably the most effective natural remedy for bruising is the homeopathic product, arnica ointment. For extensive bruising this is best backed up by the use of arnica tablets as well. Essential oils can be applied via a cold compress. To a bowl of cold water add:

- 5 drops fennel
- 5 drops lavender

Lavender also has the advantage of being suitable to apply to broken skin where arnica ointment would otherwise be contraindicated.

Burns

Lavender oil is extremely effective in treating burns. Apply immediately to the affected area, either neat or mixed with aloe gel. Aloe gel comes from the aloe plant of North America and is traditionally applied to burns directly from the plant. It is very cooling and soothing and can be obtained from branches of The Body Shop or healthfood stores. Use:

- 5ml aloe gel
- 5 drops lavender

Apply to the burn and cover with gauze. Once the heat has gone from the burn apply the following oil to help promote healing:

- 5ml wheatgerm oil
- 5 drops lavender

Cuts

Tisserand Aromatherapy Products sell an excellent antiseptic cream containing lavender, tea-tree and eucalyptus oils. Alternatively apply lavender or tea-tree neat to the cut and cover with a piece of gauze.

Period problems

Monthly periods can come and go with little impact on a woman's daily life or they can cause a catalogue of misery either through the symptoms of PMS or through painful cramps during the period itself. Aromatherapy can be extremely helpful in helping a woman cope with this monthly occurrence though if symptoms are prolonged or severe your doctor may refer you to a gynaecologist.

Painful periods

Essential oils massaged gently into the lower back and abdomen or applied via a hot compress can greatly ease the pain felt during a period. Most effective oils to use are:
- Marjoram
- Camomile
- Clary sage
- Lavender
- Cinnamon

Two blends for menstrual cramps – Use in a massage, in the bath or both!
- 50ml almond or grapeseed oil
- 15 drops marjoram
- 10 drops lavender
- 5 drops cinnamon

or

- 50ml almond or grapeseed
- 20 drops camomile
- 20 drops clary sage
- 10 drops lavender

Overdue periods

Sometimes a woman who normally has a regular cycle finds that her period is late. Common causes for this include overseas travel and stress. There are a group of essential oils, known as emmenagogues, which promote and regularise menstrual flow and these can be useful in such a situation. Obviously these must *not* be used if there is any chance that you might be pregnant. Oils to use include:

- Clary sage
- Fennel
- Rosemary
- Marjoram

A *bath* or *massage* oil for a late period

- 50ml grapeseed oil
- 15 drops clary sage
- 15 drops rosemary
- 10 drops fennel

Pre-menstrual syndrome

It is estimated that up to 90 per cent of women suffer from PMS at some time in their lives. Symptoms vary widely from slight irritability to extreme emotional disturbance which can disrupt everyday life and relationships. Physical symptoms include fluid retention, breast tenderness and headaches. Research is currently being undertaken into the effects of diet on PMS and much has been written about the benefits of dietary supplements such as evening primrose oil and vitamin B6. If your symptoms are affecting your life every month it may be worth considering a visit to a nutritionist or other health practitioner. Aromatherapy can provide excellent back-up treatment, either self-administered or through an aromatherapist. As symptoms can vary widely I have suggested oils which have an affinity with the female reproductive system as the best general oils to choose. Refer to complaints under other headings as appropriate. These oils are:

- Rose
- Camomile
- Lavender
- Geranium
- Bergamot
- Juniper

Two bath oils for PMS – Some women become tearful, miserable and lose self-esteem before a period; others become irritable and angry. The first of these blends is designed as a pick-me-up, the second as calming oil.

- 50ml grapeseed oil
- 20 drops bergamot
- 20 drops geranium
- 10 drops lavender

- 50ml grapeseed oil
- 20 drops camomile
- 20 drops lavender
- 10 drops rose

Massage oil for fluid retention – Use firm upward strokes to apply this oil concentrating on the legs. Start a few days before the symptoms usually occur and continue every day until your period starts. It is beneficial to change the blend after a couple of months. (See entry under cellulite for other suggestions.)

- 50ml almond oil
- 15 drops geranium
- 10 drops juniper
- 5 drops bergamot

Skin irritation
Aromatherapy is particularly useful in treating skin conditions as it is nearly always applied topically. For general skin-care recipes see under skin-care section on pages 82–89.

Eczema
The underlying causes of eczema are still not fully understood

and treatment can vary greatly. It is always advisable to see an aromatherapist who will discuss the condition in detail before recommending suitable oils and who may in turn refer you to another practitioner or your GP. Self-help is most appropriate when the condition is less severe and occurs occasionally in isolated areas of the body.

Soothng skin cream – Choose an unfragranced cream or lotion that suits your skin.
- 15ml cream or lotion
- 2 drops camomile
- 2 drops lavender

If no irritation occurs increase the strength up to a maximum of 10 drops of essential oil.

Sunburn
Sunburn is a radiation burn and is therefore a serious condition which should be prevented. Always use a high factor sun cream, wear a hat and other protective clothes and avoid the midday sun. Be particularly vigilant on overcast or breezy days – the sun's rays are still present even though it may not feel that hot. Always protect babies and children. If you do get burnt the best oils to use are:
- Camomile
- Lavender
- Neroli

A cooling bath – If the sunburn covers a large area of skin then take the heat out of the burn in a cool bath. Fill a bath with cool but not too cold water and add:
- 3 drops camomile
- 3 drops lavender

Repeat as often as possible until the redness subsides.

A soothing skin gel – This is ideal for isolated areas of sunburn including the face.

- 5ml aloe gel
- 5 drops camomile

Apply as often as required.

An after-sun lotion – Once the heat has gone from the sunburnt area, aid skin repair by making your own lotion.
- 50ml unfragranced body lotion
- 5ml wheatgerm oil
- 15 drops lavender
- 15 drops neroli

Alternatively try any of the oils recommended for dry or dehydrated skin on page 83.

Stings and bites
Nettle stings and insect bites can be extremely itchy and uncomfortable. Soothe the area with the following:
- 5ml aloe gel
- 5 drops camomile

AROMATHERAPY FOR STRESS AND TENSION

It is extremely hard to avoid stressful situations in our modern way of living. Sitting in a traffic jam late for an important meeting, distracting an enthusiastic toddler intent on playing with your friend's prized ornaments, listening to your neighbours' noisy lawnmower when you would love to listen to the cricket in peace – all these things have the potential to wind you up if you let them. It is easier to learn to deal with stressful situations than to avoid them, and if you find you often feel uptight, a short course in stress management could really help. Others ways to help yourself are listed at the end of this chapter under the heading 'Relaxation'. Aromatherapy baths at home can also be a wonderful way of relieving stress and tension especially if you turn them into a ritual, maybe playing calming music or lighting a few candles.

It goes without saying that in more serious cases of stress it is always advisable to seek help from a professional therapist, be they a counsellor, aromatherapist or doctor. Prolonged stress can be a major factor in aggravating many physical illnesses from heart problems to skin complaints. Prevention is better than cure, so take active steps to keep yourself as relaxed as possible.

There are very many essential oils which can be of use in dealing with stress. The symptoms of stress manifest themselves in many different ways. Some of us become depressed and lethargic while others get irritable and angry. Below I've listed some of the most useful essential oils either as relaxing or uplifting (though some appear in both lists as they tend to have a balancing effect) and then made some suggestions for blends for use in specific situations. However, the possibilities in this area are limitless so read the individual description for the oils and experiment for yourself.

Relaxing oils	Uplifting oils
Camomile	Basil
Clary sage	Bergamot
Frankincense	Cinnamon
Geranium	Geranium
Lavender	Grapefruit
Neroli	Juniper
Petitgrain	Lime
Rose	Mandarin
Sandalwood	Orange
Ylang Ylang	Rosemary

All the following suggestions are designed for use in the bath and should be added to 50ml grapeseed oil unless otherwise stated.

Home from work blends
Whatever your daytime activity there comes a time when you just want to switch off, even if all you want to do next is go to bed. If you've been surrounded by other people all day at work and on your journey home then clear your mind with:
- 20 drops geranium
- 20 drops juniper
- 10 drops orange

When you can't seem to forget the day's problems and keep
going over the same things in your mind, try:
- 20 drops clary sage
- 20 drops lavender
- 10 drops basil

If you're angry and irritable or upset over events of the day
then relax with:
- 20 drops camomile
- 20 drops lavender
- 10 drops rose

Oils to promote a good night's sleep
For a general night-time sedative it is hard to beat the
combination of:
- 20 drops lavender
- 15 drops camomile
- 15 drops sandalwood

If the sleeplessness has anything to do with fear then try:
- 20 drops bergamot
- 20 drops ylang ylang
- 10 drops lavender

Anxiety over forthcoming events
Use either of these blends in the time preceding a big event, be
it an exam, driving test or public appearance. The first
is particularly good for helping with butterflies in the
tummy:
- 20 drops neroli
- 20 drops petitgrain
- 10 drops orange

This blend helps to calm the breathing to produce a medita-
tive state:
- 20 drops frankincense
- 20 drops lavender
- 10 drops orange

If mental clarity is needed immediately before an event then try rubbing the following blend into the temples and other pulse points:

- 15ml almond oil
- 5 drops rosemary
- 1 drop mandarin
- 1 drop lime

Pick-me-up blends

If you are feeling down and lethargic then too relaxing a blend of oils may make you feel worse. The following blends are calming and uplifting at the same time. The first is very feminine:

- 20 drops geranium
- 20 drops rose
- 10 drops lavender

The second blend has a fresh fragrance:

- 20 drops bergamot
- 20 drops petitgrain
- 10 drops orange

Oils for fatigue and exhaustion

Working long hours or suffering from some form of illness can be very stressful and leave you lacking energy. After illness try:

- 20 drops bergamot
- 10 drops grapefruit
- 10 drops lime

As a general tonic use:

- 20 drops rosemary
- 15 drops mandarin
- 5 drops cinnamon

AROMATHERAPY AND SKIN CARE

From the early beginnings of modern aromatherapy, essential oils have been used to promote healthy skin. Many products are now available to buy ready made but it is also nice to experiment with your own blends. A good daily skin-care routine consists of thorough cleansing followed by the use of a skin freshener and then a product to moisturize. Weekly treatments include face masks and scrubs. Essential oils really come into their own in the latter part of this routine as cleansing products have only a short contact time with the skin before they are removed. Many of the oils have a balancing effect on the skin so appear in the lists for more than one skin type.

Dry skin

Dry skin can either lack sebum, the skin's own natural oil, or be dehydrated or often both. It can feel tight especially after washing and though it has a fine appearance in youth it has a tendency to wrinkle more easily if not well cared for. The best oils to use include:

- Rose
- Camomile
- Neroli
- Sandalwood
- Lavender

Cleansing

Use a naturally based cream or lotion as soap and other washes can dry the skin further. Apply the product directly to the skin and remove with damp cotton wool.

Freshening

Use a mild skin freshener or make up the following:

- 100ml rosewater
- 2.5ml vodka
- 3 drops geranium
- 3 drops rose

The vodka in this recipe is used to dissolve the essential oils before adding the flower water. Rosewater is available from most good chemists. Also look out for other flower waters such as camomile and lavender which are available from some of the specialist suppliers.

Moisturizing

Any of the essential oils listed above can be added to your normal daily moisturizer though one of the most effective ways of treating dry skin is using an oil at night-time. Try the following recipes:

For dry skin with thread veins

- 25ml almond oil
- 20ml avocado oil or peach kernel oil
- 5ml wheatgerm oil
- 15 drops camomile
- 15 drops rose

For dry and dehydrated skin

- 25ml almond oil
- 20ml avocado or peach kernel oil
- 5ml wheatgerm oil
- 15 drops lavender
- 15 drops sandalwood

Apply this oil to the skin while it is still damp from the freshener to lock the moisture in.

Treatments

Face masks are popular weekly treatments and can be either commercially prepared or based on natural raw ingredients. Find a good natural beauty book and have some fun with the recipes, adding a few drops of essential oil to make them even more effective. Alternatively use a facial scrub once a week to gently remove the dead cells from the surface of the skin leaving it feeling smoother and looking brighter. Always moisturize after using a treatment.

Oily skin

Oily skin is caused by an over-production of sebum and while it seems to age somewhat better than dry skin it can be prone to spots, blackheads and, in teenage years, acne. If the acne is

severe, it is important to consult a professional aromatherapist, doctor or other practitioner who may also be able to
offer other advice. Essential oils to use are:

- Bergamot
- Lavender
- Tea-tree
- Clary sage

Cleansing
Skin-care products for this type can often be quite harsh,
stripping the oil from the skin so effectively that more is
produced to compensate. Deep cleansing with a cream or
lotion is important if make-up is worn and can always be
followed by a mild face wash to make the skin feel squeaky
clean.

Freshening
Toners based on alcohol not only remove the excess oil but
can also remove too much water leaving the skin with flaky
patches. The following is a recipe for a mild skin freshener:

- 100ml orange flower water
- 2.5ml vodka
- 3 drops bergamot
- 3 drops lavender

The orange flower water can be obtained from the chemist.
For a slightly more astringent effect, replace some of the
orange flower water with witch hazel.

Moisturizing
Even oily skin needs protection from the elements. Including
essential oils in a moisturizer will help to fight the bacteria
which contribute to the formation of spots and acne. Add
essential oils to a light daytime moisturizer or try:

- 20ml aloe gel
- 10ml wheatgerm oil
- 3 drops lavender
- 2 drops clary sage

- 2 drops tea-tree

At night-time try using jojoba oil as a base. It has a chemical composition similar to that of sebum and is reputed to help balance the skin's production of oil.
- 50ml jojoba oil
- 10 bergamot
- 10 drops clary sage
- 10 drops lavender

If this feels too greasy then mix equal parts of this blend and aloe gel together and apply directly to the skin.

Treatments
Using a face scrub twice a week will help prevent the blocked pores that can lead to spots. However, if the skin already has red spots with pus, the scrubbing will only make things worse. Instead try steaming the face including any of the above essential oils in the water.

Normal or combination skin
You may be one of those lucky people whose skin is neither too oily nor too dry or, more likely, you will have skin which is oily in parts and dry in others. The classic combination is to have dry cheeks with an oily strip across the forehead and down the nose and chin. You can use a combination of products on different parts of the face or you can use oils which have a balancing effect such as:
- Geranium
- Lavender
- Ylang ylang
- Sandalwood

Use your normal cleansing products and try the following blends. As a freshener make:
- 100ml lavender water (the pure flower water not the cologne) or orange flower water

- 2.5ml vodka
- 3 drops geranium
- 3 drops ylang ylang

As a night-time treatment use:
- 25ml almond oil
- 20ml jojoba oil
- 5ml wheatgerm oil
- 10 drops lavender
- 10 drops sandalwood
- 10 drops ylang ylang

Sensitive skin

This term can be misleading as each person may be sensitive to different things. In general stick to very mild and gentle products and if in doubt try any new product on the inside of the elbow first. Wait 24 hours and if no reaction has occurred then try the product on the face. The oils listed under the section for dry skin are all very mild oils and would be suitable to use. If the skin is red or sore try the blends listed under skin irritation.

Cellulite

Essential oils make great facial skin-care products but can also benefit the skin on the rest of the body too. One body condition that is worth further mention is cellulite. Use the blends above as bath or body massage products replacing some of the more expensive carrier oils for grapeseed oil.

It is thought than as many as 80 per cent of western women have cellulite to some degree yet the medical profession tends to view it as something created by the beauty industry as a way of selling more products. It affects women almost exclusively and some people claim that it is a normal condition which women have had over the centuries. It is only modern media pressure that has led women to see it as unattractive and therefore a problem. Holistic practitioners would tend to disagree, believing instead that too many toxins in the body are a major contributory factor. These toxins cause the walls of the fat cells found underneath the surface of the skin to become thicker, locking in the toxic deposits and water. Activity of the hormone oestrogen is also thought to play a part in the formation of cellulite, explaining why it is a female condition.

Cellulite is most commonly found on the thighs, hips, buttocks and occasionally the upper arms and makes the skin look lumpy under the surface. A holistic approach is the most successful in the treatment of cellulite, including diet and exercise as well as massage with essential oils. A serious case of cellulite will benefit from a series of treatments from an aromatherapist who will discuss with you the underlying causes and use a specific type of massage to help the condition. You can help to diminish the cellulite by following the five-step plan below.

Diet
This is not necessarily a slimming diet but a cleansing one (see under nutrition later in this chapter). A short fast often gives this process a kick start.

Water
Drink at least six glasses a day to help cleanse the cells of toxins.

Exercise
Aerobic exercise helps to stimulate the lymphatic system which helps the body to rid itself of waste products. Swimming or cycling seem to be more effective than high impact aerobics, and stretching and toning exercises also help.

Skin brushing
Daily dry skin brushing is a wonderful way of helping the body to rid itself of toxins. Use a natural bristle brush and always work upwards towards the heart.

Aromatherapy massage

Use firm upward strokes on the legs concentrating on the tops and sides of the thighs. An aromatherapist will show you how to do this effectively. You can also use a massage mitt with the essential oil blends. The best oils to use include:

- Geranium
- Juniper
- Fennel
- Rosemary
- Black Pepper
- Lemon

Massage daily after a bath or shower alternating the oils to retain their effectiveness. Two blends to use are:

- 50ml grapeseed oil
- 15 drops geranium
- 10 drops rosemary
- 5 drops black pepper

or

- 50ml grapeseed oil
- 10 drops juniper
- 5 drops fennel
- 5 drops lemon

AROMATHERAPY FOR MOTHER AND BABY

Pregnancy and early motherhood can be an exciting, exhausting yet truly amazing time in a woman's life. It can also be a time of ups and downs, the initial excitement of discovering that you're pregnant could be followed by weeks of nausea, the joy and wonderment at seeing your new-born baby may be accompanied by months of sleepless nights. It can also have its share of stress, whether it it is caused by the wait for test results during pregnancy, the feelings of helplessness when you have a colicky baby, the decision whether or not to return to work or the labour itself.

Aromatherapy can be a wonderful way to ease some of

these stresses and help some physical conditions as well. Yet pick up any book on aromatherapy and warnings on using essential oils abound. Sometimes you find an oil that is recommended in one book is not advised in another so you decide not to bother at all. Stick to the oils listed below and you'll be fine, but if you need further reassurance then speak to an aromatherapist who will put your mind at rest.

Pregnancy

In the following list I've concentrated on the oils that are universally thought to be safe to use during pregnancy. Many others are recommended in other books and if you feel confident to try them then that's fine. Even with my reduced list of oils there is still a choice of 12 and plenty of scope for experimentation. Try to vary your choice of oils on a regular basis, and as skin can become more sensitive make the dilutions lower than usual.

- Bergamot
- Frankincense
- Grapefruit
- Mandarin
- Neroli
- Orange
- Petitgrain
- Sandalwood
- Tea-tree
- Ylang ylang

The next oils can also be safely used after the first three months of pregnancy:
- Camomile
- Lavender

Backache

As the pregnancy progresses the additional weight of the baby can put a strain on the lower back. Correct posture can help enormously – tuck your pelvis under and try not to stick your bump out more than necessary – as can a back massage given by a partner or friend. At this stage it will probably be uncomfortable to lie down for a massage. Try sitting the wrong way round on a dining chair (one without arms), place a cushion on the back of the chair and rest your arms and head on this. Alternatively make yourself comfortable on some large floor cushions. Use this blend for massage or in the bath.

- 50ml almond oil
- 8 drops camomile
- 8 drops lavender
- 4 drops orange

Emotional effects of pregnancy

In addition to the physical symptoms that may accompany pregnancy, it can be an intensely emotional time as well. It is important to remain as calm as possible and make every effort to keep up your strength – you'll need all the energy you can muster for the labour and following months of motherhood. Try the following oils in the bath or for a massage.

A deeply relaxing bedtime oil

- 50ml grapeseed oil
- 8 drops frankincense
- 8 drops sandalwood
- 4 drops orange

An oil for anxiety as the birth approaches

- 50ml grapeseed oil
- 8 drops neroli
- 8 drops petitgrain
- 4 drops orange

High blood pressure

Your blood pressure will be monitored regularly throughout the pregnancy and if it does rise you may be kept under close medical supervision. The following blend can help you remain calm and deal with the anxiety that this may bring.

- 50ml grapeseed oil
- 8 drops bergamot

- 8 drops ylang ylang
- 4 drops lavender

Morning sickness
Most oils indicated for nausea are not recommended so try fennel tea instead.

Oedema
Slight puffiness of the fingers, legs and feet is normal during pregnancy. However, if swelling is excessive seek medical advice to rule out any more serious conditions. Resting with the feet higher than the legs can help. Massage the legs with smooth upward movements or use the following oil in the bath:
- 50ml almond or grapeseed oil
- 8 drops grapefruit
- 8 drops lavender
- 4 drops mandarin

Prevention of stretch marks
Daily massage of the tummy, breasts and upper legs with this blend of essential oils will keep the skin soft and supple and help to prevent the formation of stretch marks. Massage on the abdomen is fine as long as it is done gently in clockwise circular movements. It can be enjoyable for the baby as well.
- 25ml almond oil
- 25ml wheatgerm oil
- 15 drops mandarin
- 15 drops neroli

Tiredness
It's hard to describe the overwhelming tiredness that many women feel in the early months of pregnancy. It comes at a time when you don't look pregnant and you may not have told anybody yet so you get little sympathy, especially at work! The following blend makes a cheery and refreshing morning bath.
- 50ml grapeseed oil

- 10 drops bergamot
- 10 drops petitgrain
- 5 drops grapefruit

Labour

As the pregnancy draws to a close some women can't wait for the birth to happen. Others get more and more nervous as the due date approaches. However you feel it is important to be as well informed as possible by attending ante-natal classes. You may have your heart set on a particular type of birth but it is wise to keep as open a mind as possible as no one can predict exactly how they will cope once the labour begins. Any of the oils listed under pregnancy can be used for massage during labour. Pick your favourite oils and make up a blend beforehand. These additional oils are some of the most widely used and beneficial to use during labour.

- Jasmine
- Lavender
- Clary sage

A blend to prepare for labour

It is well worth investing in some jasmine as it is the supreme oil for labour. Take the following bath daily for a week before your expected due date to help prepare the uterus, and use in baths or massage at the onset of labour.

- 50ml grapeseed oil
- 15 drops jasmine
- 15 drops lavender

Clary sage can be used in place of jasmine if you prefer. Also use this blend to help expel the placenta quickly.

Other remedies to help you through labour

Certain homeopathic remedies can be of great help during labour and are best recommended by a professional homeopath. Alternatively a great self-help treatment is to take

Rescue Remedy (see page 98 for more information on the Bach Flower remedies).

After the birth

The emotional ups and downs which follow the birth can be quite bewildering; tears of joy one minute followed by moments of panic as an overwhelming sense of responsibility hits you. Throughout the pregnancy many women focus on the birth and feel ill prepared for life with a new baby. Suddenly any time to yourself feels like a complete luxury but it is worth using this time to recuperate, relax and try to regain your strength. Refer to the previous sections to find blends which are most appropriate to the way you are feeling. Aromatherapy can also aid your recovery on a physical level too.

A bath for healing stitches

Add 5 or 6 drops of lavender oil directly to the bath water. Bathe as many times as is practical for the first week. It is best to avoid the use of any carrier oil in the water until the stitches heal. Taking the homeopathic remedy of arnica can help with any bruising (as well as helping to recover from the trauma of labour). Take hourly for the first day then take two or three times a day for the next few days as necessary.

Helping the uterus contract

After the birth the uterus contracts to its pre-pregnancy size. This process can be felt as sharp contractions known as after-pains. Breast feeding helps this process and you can also massage the abdomen using:
- 50ml almond oil
- 20 drops jasmine

Breast feeding

There are so many advantages to breast feeding that it is certainly worth a good try for at least the early weeks. If you have problems contact a breast feeding counsellor. Some essential oils can be of help too.

Promoting the milk supply

For the first few days of life a baby is nourished by colostrum. The milk supply comes in after this and drinking fennel tea can be helpful. If you prefer you can use fennel oil in a massage blend.

Engorged breasts

If the breasts become painfully full, try a cold compress of peppermint oil to help ease the discomfort.

Cracked nipples

The most effective treatment for sore or cracked nipples is calendula cream. Apply after each feed and remove any traces before the next one.

Babies and toddlers

Essential oils can be used on babies from birth provided they are well diluted. This means using one drop only in each teaspoon of oil. Never put essential oils neat into a baby's bath. It is also best to stick to the mildest oils in the early days, introducing other oils as your child grows older. The best oils to use are:

- Camomile
- Lavender
- Mandarin
- Rose
- Sandalwood

Aromatherapy can be used for some of the physical complaints suffered by babies and can also help when they (and you!) are feeling fractious. A friend of mine once described her baby as a barometer of her emotions and it is very true that babies do pick up so easily on our moods. So join in with your baby's calming bath, you're probably in need of it as much as he or she is. There is one 'baby blend' of oils that is useful in so many situations that it is worth having a bottle made up ready:

- 50ml almond oil
- 5 drops camomile
- 5 drops lavender

Many babies also respond well to massage. You don't need to be trained to do this. Just use gentle stroking movements and follow your intuition. Some massage books have good sequences for baby massage which are nice to follow but don't be worried if your baby won't lie in the positions suggested. Do what your baby enjoys and leave the rest out. Always make sure the room is warm enough before you start and make sure you are comfortable too. Stop whenever one of you has had enough thus keeping the whole experience a pleasurable one for both of you.

Colds and coughs
If your baby has a stuffy nose then try putting a drop of lavender and a drop of eucalyptus on a hanky and put it under the sheet at night. For a cough gently rub a mixture of the following blend on the baby's chest and upper back.
- 50ml almond oil
- 5 drops lavender
- 5 drops sandalwood

Colic
Every baby book differs on the cause of 'colic' which by most is described as crying incessantly, often in the late afternoon or evening. If your baby is normally cheerful at other times of the day then a visit to your doctor will reassure you that nothing is seriously wrong and that it is a phase that will pass. Gently massaging your baby, if he or she will let you, may help to calm them down and if it doesn't then at least you will feel as if you are doing something to help. Use the blend given above.

Cradle cap
This is like a crust that forms on the scalp and is completely harmless to the baby. You can help to soften the scales by gently applying almond oil on its own or, if you prefer, use the

blend above. Warm the oil in your hands before applying. Another suggestion is to try chickweed cream which you should find in a healthfood shop.

Dry skin

If your baby has dry skin then it is best to avoid using bubble baths or soaps, even ones which are specially designed for infants. Use the blend above instead. This can also be used for all-over massage.

Nappy rash

Nappy rash can appear quickly and sometimes takes a while to clear up. One of the best pieces of advice is to keep the baby out of a nappy for as much of the day as possible, which is fine at home but more problematic if you are out and about all day. You can help soothe the skin by using the baby blend in the bath. Before putting on a nappy use some calendula cream or some Rescue Remedy cream.

Teething

Once your baby has passed the colic stage it can seem like all bouts of crying or fractiousness are attributed to teething. I always found it difficult to know if this was the case but signs to look for include redness on the cheeks and the baby constantly biting on hard objects. Essential oils, even if diluted, should never be put in the mouth but can be rubbed on the cheeks and jaw line. Try using camomile diluted in almond oil.

Wind

Gentle massage on the tummy in a clockwise direction can be helpful to release trapped wind. You can use the general baby blend or use mandarin diluted in almond oil instead.

Children

As your children get older they can continue to benefit from aromatherapy. You can use the suggestions made elsewhere in this book, just make sure that you keep the dilutions low and avoid using any of the oils that are not recommended for sensitive skin. Children will often love to be massaged and as a bonus they will soon want to give you a massage in return.

COMPLEMENTARY HOME TREATMENTS

In addition to aromatherapy there are some other treatments and techniques which you can use at home to keep yourself in good shape. Details of these are listed below.

Bach Flower Remedies

The Bach flower remedies comprise a system of 38 remedies prepared from the flowers of wild plants, trees and bushes. They are not used directly for physical complaints but rather for the mental state behind them. The belief is that not only do negative states of mind, such as fear, hopelessness and irritability, hinder recovery from illness but they are in fact the primary cause of ill health and disease. Dr Edward Bach was a Welsh doctor, who gave up his practice in 1930 to develop his series of remedies which work on a very subtle level, allowing patients to find peace and harmony and thereby heal themselves. The difference between flower remedies and essential oils is that essential oils work on physical, mental and emotional levels simultaneously. Some aromatherapists use the remedies to back up their treatment with essential oils and give clients a bottle of prepared remedy to take home. However the instructions and literature on the Bach remedies are self-explanatory and they are thus ideal for self-help. There are some good books around and many people find that reading about the principles of the 38 remedies helps them discover personality traits or negative states of mind.

The remedies are roughly seen as being of two different groups. The first group of 'type' remedies are said to define the basic fundamental nature of a person. Most people can identify with a 'type' remedy which will have both positive and negative states. If you have a tendency to display the negative traits of a certain remedy, taking it will help you move back to its positive state. Other remedies are seen as 'helpers' which are used to back-up 'type' remedies or to give help at particular moments in time. For example, agrimony, a 'type' remedy, is for people who tend to hide worries behind a brave face, whereas walnut is a 'helper' used for times of change or transition, be it puberty, marriage or a new job.

The remedies are available from some chemists and many healthfood shops. They come with a free leaflet, giving instructions on use and a brief description of each remedy. You may want to start just with this and move on to more detailed books later. The remedies are completely safe, with no side-effects. You cannot choose the 'wrong' remedy, if your body does not need one of the ones you take it simply will not use it.

Nutrition

'You are what you eat' is a phrase that is widely used these days, yet one that many people pay little attention to. Though there is a general trend towards healthier eating, our super-market shelves are still stocked with sugar, salt and additive laden foods with little nutritional value. The aromatherapist will probably ask about your diet during the case history and in some cases it may be suggested that you make radical changes in your diet to supplement your treatment.

Conditions which are aggravated by eating the wrong foods include arthritis, acne, catarrh and many stress related problems. A lot of work has been done on diet and arthritis sufferers and there are some excellent books around full of case histories to show that dietary change really can help. The diets may be strict and you need to be committed to follow them, but the results can be dramatic. Teenagers with acne have notoriously bad diets, snacking on crisps, sweets and fizzy drinks. They may find it hard, but a change in diet is really essential. Catarrh sufferers will benefit from cutting down on mucous forming foods such as dairy and wheat products and for all stress related conditions a reduction in the intake of stimulants, tea, coffee, alcohol and some food additives, can be important. Even if you have no particular health problems at present, a good diet is a good form of preventative healthcare.

When we talk about changing our diet, most people think only about the things they will have to cut out. I prefer to concentrate on all the new things they have never thought of trying. So you have to cut down on tea and coffee, but there is a huge range of herbal teas to experiment with these days. Instead of the staple bread, rice and pasta, try grains like millet, buckwheat, bulgar and couscous. Meat intake can be reduced by increasing the amount of pulses, nuts and seeds we eat. The basic rules for good nutrition are as follows. Try to avoid pre-packaged foods as much as possible, replacing them with fresh foods. If you do eat canned or packet food, choose ones without additives, sugar or salt. Eat plenty of fresh fruit and vegetables, organically grown is best but not practical for most people – wash it well instead. If you eat meat, cut right down on red meat, replacing it with lean white meat, or better still eat more fish. Vegetarianism is fine, but do not go overboard on the dairy produce. Try to keep your diet as varied as possible with plenty of different grains, pulses, nuts and seeds. Coffee is best avoided, but if you cannot give it up, cut down to a couple of cups a day and keep tea intake down as well. If you still want to drink alcohol, stick to wine and try diluting it with spring water.

Once you have discovered how good it feels to eat well, you might want to take it a stage further and try the occasional fast. This does not mean cutting out all food but could instead involve just eating fruit and vegetables for a few days or just drinking grape juice and spring water. On page 112 I have given the address of an organization that produce books and leaflets on diets but if you are in any doubt or if you have any medical condition, check with your doctor first before fasting.

Nutritional supplements
In theory we should be able to get all our requirements for vitamins and minerals from our food. In practice few of us have a perfect diet and environmental factors, such as

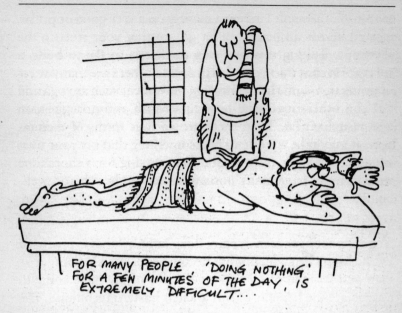

FOR MANY PEOPLE, 'DOING NOTHING' FOR A FEW MINUTES OF THE DAY, IS EXTREMELY DIFFICULT....

pollution, increase our need for vitamins. If you feel as though you need to take some supplements but are overwhelmed by the array of bottles and packets in the healthfood shop, ask your aromatherapist for some advice. He or she may be able to suggest a reputable brand of multi-vitamins/minerals (some are laden with sugar and additives) or, if you need more specific advice, recommend a nutritional consultant. Many conditions these days are being treated by high dosage supplementation, though this should always be undertaken under the guidance of a trained nutritionist.

Relaxation

For most of us, relaxation is sitting in front of the television, reading a good book, taking a long walk or enjoying a game of squash. Though these are all good forms of stress release or of switching off from the daily grind of work, the emphasis is still on *doing* something rather than simply *being*. We live in a world which puts ever increasing importance on making things happen, rather than letting things happen, and for many people 'doing nothing' even for a few minutes a day is extremely difficult. Having a massage is a very good opportunity to lie for an hour and let go, putting your trust in the therapist. Taking this one step further is to try to build a relaxation spot into your daily routine. There are many ways of doing this, some incorporating movement such as yoga and t'ai chi, others involving techniques such as autosuggestion and visualization. Then there are various forms of meditation. It may take a while to find something that fits your own lifestyle, but there is no doubt that relaxing for a short time each day can have many positive effects on health and well-being.

Yoga

Yoga is no longer seen as something 'cranky' that is practised by the hippy brigade, but has become enormously popular as men and women of all ages and walks of life have come to appreciate the benefits of this ancient Eastern technique. The most common form of yoga taught and practised in Britain is hatha yoga. This involves a system of stretching postures or *asanas* which exercise all parts of the body, keeping muscles well-tuned and stimulating the circulation. In addition to this you will learn breathing exercises, or pranayama, which are wonderfully calming and revitalizing, and some form of meditation technique. You can teach yourself yoga from a book, though most people prefer to join a class and learn with a group of others from a qualified teacher. You will then find it easier to practise at home. Most adult education centres run yoga evening classes or maybe a local community centre runs drop-in classes where you turn up and pay week by week.

T'ai chi chuan

Though not as well known as yoga at present, t'ai chi is becoming increasingly popular. Its roots are in ancient China and it can be used as a form of self-defence, though in the West it is most often used as a form of exercise to relax the mind and body. When practising t'ai chi you learn what is known as a form, which for beginners consists of about 50 different postures linked together by slow, gentle, flowing movements. Like yoga, it exercises muscles, improves circulation and balances energy levels. Again, it can be practised by people of any age. All you need is a small space and you can even practise in the office at lunchtime for ten minutes or so. It is important though to find a good teacher to learn the basics from, and then you can practise daily.

Autosuggestion and autogenic training

Autosuggestion is something we do subconsciously all the time. We talk ourselves into feeling warm because the sun is out, even though there might be a cold breeze. Using this idea we can consciously talk ourselves into a state of relaxation by sitting or lying quietly and repeating slowly to ourselves words like 're-lax' or 'he-avy'.

A more sophisticated version of this technique is known as autogenic training or AT and is a method of deep relaxation and greater self-awareness. It can be practised in either a sitting or a lying position and involves persuading various parts of the body to generate their own sensations. You begin by turning your attention to one part of the body and saying, for example, 'my right arm is heavy', repeating this until your arm really does feel heavy and then moving on to another part of your body. You then progress to thinking yourself warm. Next you 'think' your heart beat calm and register your breathing as slow and deep, your abdomen (solar plexus) warm, and your forehead cool. At the end of the exercise you return to the world with the phrase 'I am refreshed and alert.'

The exercises should involve an attitude of 'passive concentration' where you say the phrase then observe what sensations or emotions you become aware of. Some people find this system quite hard to use on their own at first and so use a taped sequence, either made themselves or bought ready-made. Though obviously using a tape is not quite the same as autosuggestion, as you cannot work at your own pace, it is still a very useful relaxation aid.

Progressive relaxation

This is a simpler technique than AT (see above) and can be practised easily at home with no tuition necessary. It involves putting a group of muscles into a state of tension, then letting

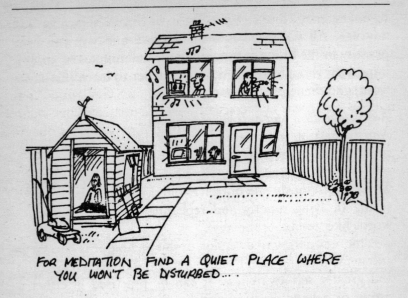

FOR MEDITATION FIND A QUIET PLACE WHERE
YOU WON'T BE DISTURBED....

go and feeling the different sensation. You usually begin at
your toes, working right up your face, finally trying to clear
your mind of all thoughts. Again you can use a tape (or a
friend) to talk you through the sequence.

Meditation

Many people think of meditation as something practised by
Buddhist monks or various religious sects. This is not so and
the many forms of meditation can be extremely beneficial for
overcoming anxiety, releasing tension and refreshing the
mind. When practised, meditation can produce what is
known as a *hypometabolic* (very relaxed) state of body,
where your heart beat slows down, blood pressure drops and
breathing becomes slower and shallower. Your mind
switches to a state of 'relaxed wakefulness'. This state can be
more restful and constructive than sleep. Meditation can
either be 'taught' as in transcendental meditation (TM) or
learnt at home following a few simple guidelines. In TM you
will go to an introductory talk, then have several individual
sessions with an instructor where you will be given your own
personal mantra or chant, to use when you meditate. While

some people find that they need to learn the technique in order to have the will power to practise at home, others find they can manage quite well by following these four basic conditions. First is finding a quiet place where you will not be disturbed, second is sitting or lying in a relaxed position. You then need to focus on a constant mental stimulus. This could be auditory, a sound or a word or phrase repeated either silently or out loud, or a visual image, either an actual object or a mental picture. Finally, you need to adopt a passive attitude, that is not working too hard at achieving anything, and if thoughts come in, just note them and return to the technique. Meditation like this is known as concentration or contemplation and is the type most commonly practised in the West. At much deeper levels of meditation the practitioner will completely forget the self and leave behind both body and mind as he or she transcends to a higher state of being.

7
THE FUTURE
OF AROMATHERAPY

Interest in aromatherapy has grown enormously in the last ten years and as this trend continues, there are likely to be many changes and developments. Below is a brief discussion of how aromatheraphy may progress in the future.

BEAUTY PRODUCTS AND PERFUMES

Many manufacturers of cosmetics and even some of the large fragrance houses have jumped on the aromatherapy band-wagon and are marketing products containing essential oils. Professionals in the field of aromatherapy are in two minds as to the merits of this. Some feel that it is trivializing the more serious side of aromatherapy, while others think that by drawing the public's attention to aromatherapy in this form, some people are more likely to explore the topic further. Sometimes the so-called aromatherapy oils on sale are synthetic and not natural oils, though it is often difficult for an untrained nose to tell the difference. If you are interested in aromatherapy beauty products, some of the suppliers' addresses, who deal with mail order, are given on page 112.

MEDICAL (OR CLINICAL) AROMATHERAPY

Turning to the other end of the spectrum, there is a growing interest in the medical uses of aromatherapy. At present there are very few practitioners in Britain who use essential oils to treat infectious or organic diseases. Those who do are either herbalists or orthodox doctors, both of whom are legally able to diagnose disease and prescribe medication. The story is slightly different in France, where most people have followed the same path as Dr Jean Valnet and his way of using essential oils (see page 4). It is now possible to undertake courses in scientific aromatherapy in Britain but there is some debate as to whether it is safe to teach non-medically qualified people about the medical uses of essential oils. Perhaps one hope for the future would be to have an aromatherapy course similar to that taken by medical herbalists, covering all aspects of aromatherapy including clinical diagnosis as well as holistic pratice.

HOLISTIC AROMATHERAPY

This book has covered the use of aromatherapy in what could be termed as its holistic form – looking at the whole person and treating the underlying causes of disease. It often deals with psychosomatic illness, but considering that even the BMA agrees that a high proportion of disease could be classified as such, then it is no less important than so-called clinical aromatherapy (see above). It is this type of aromatherapy that is now earning its reputation in the medical world as an effective complementary therapy. Many GPs are realizing that their patients can benefit enormously from the nurturing touch and the sympathetic ear of a qualified aromatherapist or masseur, someone who can spend more time than the allotted ten minutes in most surgeries. Indeed a GP may now refer a patient to a complementary therapist under the NHS provided they retain control of the case. Some surgeries employ an aromatherapist based on the premises for this purpose. The nursing and midwifery professions have also taken aromatherapy on board with many of them now undertaking the training. Often this is a result of working alongside aromatherapists who offer their services on a voluntary basis to treat patients on the ward. The continued exposure of the orthodox medical profession to aromatherapy can only serve to promote aromatherapists as serious healthcare professionals.

AROMATHERAPY ORGANIZATIONS COUNCIL

In 1991 the Aromatherapy Organizations Council (AOC) was formed and is now the governing body for the aromotherapy profession in the UK. It brought together the various aromatherapy associations under one umbrella and provides a collective voice through which to initiate and sustain dialogue with government, civil and medical bodies. Towards the end of 1994 it successfully organized, on behalf of the aromatherapy profession, a protest to stop the proposed licensing of essential oils under an EU directive.

The AOC has also produced a core curriculum which sets out minimum standards for all its affiliated training establishments and is currently investigating the introduction of NVQs for aromatherapists. Another key function of the AOC is to hold a database of research material and to support or sponsor research into aromatherapy where appropriate.

The AOC is a member of the British Complementary Medicine Association whose primary aim is to integrate complementary medicine in the structure of the nation's healthcare system. The formation of the AOC has been a very positive step forward for the world of aromatherapy and for the general public who can now be assured that any aromatherapist belonging to a member organization will have been trained to a set standard, will abide by a code of conduct and ethics and will be fully insured to practise. To simplify matters further it is hoped that a British Register of Aromatherapists will soon be compiled.

Affiliated to the AOC is the Aromatherapy Trades Council (ATC), a self-regulating body for the aromatherapy industry set up to raise standards and offer protection to the consumer. It promotes the responsible use of aromatherapy products and has established guidelines for safety, labelling and packaging for the aromatherapy trade.

. . . AND FINALLY

Aromatherapy is now the fastest growing therapy in the UK and is constantly gaining credibility among the medical profession and the general public. Much scientific research is being undertaken by well-respected scientists into essential oils and their effects on the body. While this research will undoubtedly give aromatherapy more kudos, we should not belittle the benefits many patients have received purely from the caring, holistic approach of complementary therapists in all fields. After all if we manage to give our clients the ability to heal themselves, the method we use is purely secondary.

USEFUL ADDRESSES

PROFESSIONAL ORGANIZATIONS

Aromatherapy Organizations Council (AOC)
The Secretary
3 Latymer Close
Braybrooke
Market Harborough
Leicester LE16 8LN

The governing body for the aromatherapy profession in the UK. They can provide a general information booklet listing the member organizations and training establishments. Please send an SAE for further details.

International Federation of Aromatherapists (IFA)
Stamford House
2–4 Chiswick High Road
London W4 1TH
Tel: 0181 742 2605

Send an sae for a list of accredited training schools or a list of IFA members. You may also join the IFA as a friend, no special qualifications needed.

TRAINING SCHOOLS

There are many colleges teaching aromatherapy and the AOC will provide a list of those which follow their core curriculum and therefore meet a minimum standard. Courses vary in duration and method of learning from part home-study courses to full-time lecture-based programmes. They will also reflect a medical, holistic or cosmetic bias in their approach.

ESSENTIAL OIL SUPPLIERS

Shops
Neal's Yard Remedies
15 Neal's Yard
Covent Garden
London WC2H 9DP
Tel: 0171 379 7222

Sells essential oils, aromatherapy products and herbal remedies. They have branches around the UK and also sell through other retail outlets. Mail order catalogue available by telephoning 01865 245436.

The Body Shop International PLC
Watersmead
Littlehampton
West Sussex BN17 6LS
Tel: 01903 731500

Sells ready blended aromatherapy products, carrier oils, aloe gel, and naturally based skin-care products. List of branches and mail order from the above address.

Ranges available through chemists and healthfood shops
Fleur Aromatherapy
Pembroke Studios
Pembroke Road
London N10 2JE
Tel: 0171 444 7424

Sells essential oils, carrier oils, starter kits, etc., through outlets and by mail order.

Tisserand Aromatherapy Products
Brighton BN3 7BA
Tel: 01273 325666

Sells essential oils and a wide range of aromatherapy products
through outlets and by mail order.

Mail Order
Eve Taylor (London Ltd)
9 Papyrus Road
Werrington Business Park
Werrington
Peterborough PE4 5BH
Tel: 01733 321101

Shirley Price Aromatherapy Limited
CW02, Essentia House
Upper Bond Street
Hinckley
Leicestershire LE10 1RS
Tel: 01455 615466

Quinessence,
Dept. AT
1 Birch Avenue
Whitwick
Leicester LE67 5GB
Tel: 01530 838358

NUTRITION

You can join either of the following organizations or send for
their book lists.

Institute of Optimum Nutrition
3 Jerdan Place
London SW6 1BE
Tel: 0171 385 7984

FURTHER READING

AROMATHERAPY

Aromatherapy, Judith Jackson (Dorling Kindersley)

Useful guide for those wishing to experiment with aromatherapy massage. Includes a good self-massage sequence.

Aromatherapy, an A to Z, Patrica Davies (C W Daniel)

Comprehensive guide to essential oils and their uses, plus many other related topics.

Aromatherapy Workbook, Shirley Price (Thorsons)

A detailed guide to aromatherapy covering information on essential oils and their application as well as a section on the chemistry of essential oils.

The Art of Aromatherapy, Robert Tisserand (C W Daniel)

An essential book for professionals and lay people alike. Background information on history and use of essential oils, plus comprehensive profiles of 24 commonly used oils.

The Directory of Essential Oils Wanda Sellar (C W Daniel)

A comprehensive guide to essential oils listing their use, chemical constituents and history set out in an easy-to-use format.

The Fragrant Pharmacy Valerie Ann Worwood (Bantam)

An interesting book written in an anecdotal style and packed with information on essential oils and their application.

MASSAGE

The Book of Massage, various authors (Ebury Press)

Comprehensive guide covering massage, shiatsu and reflexology. Plenty of illustrations, step by step instructions and authoritative advice.

The Massage Book, George Downing (Penguin)

Written in 1974, this book really describes the Esalen method of massage. It gives thorough instructions for a full body massage.

Massage Cures, Nigel Dawson and Fiona Harrold (Thorsons)

A family guide to curing common ailments with simple massage techniques. Includes good sections on pregnancy, childbirth and massage for babies and infants.

Massage for Healing and Relaxation, Carola Beresford Cooke (Arlington Books)

This is a book of a television series. Includes massage for different groups of people, from the elderly to children and babies. Includes some shiatsu and a self-massage sequence.

BACH FLOWER REMEDIES

Bach Flower Therapy, Mechfild Scheffer (Thorsons)

How to use the 38 remedies, plus a full profile of each.

Also any of the guides produced by:
The Bach Centre
Mount Vernon
Sotwell
Wallingford
Oxon OX10 0PZ
Tel: 01491 839489

JOURNALS

Aromatherapy Quarterly
Dept. AT
Ranelagh Avenue
London SW13 0BY

Index